Managing the Kidney when the Heart is Failing

George L. Bakris

Editor

Managing the Kidney when the Heart is Failing

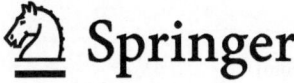 Springer

Editor
George L. Bakris
Department of Medicine
Director, ASH Comprehensive Hypertension Center
The University of Chicago Medicine
Chicago, IL, USA

This book is a compilation of selected chapters originally published in Bakris, The Kidney in Heart Failure, ISBN: 978-1-4614-3693-5

ISBN 978-1-4614-3690-4   ISBN 978-1-4614-3691-1 (eBook)
DOI 10.1007/978-1-4614-3691-1
Springer New York Heidelberg Dordrecht London

Library of Congress Control Number: 2012940204

Printed on acid-free paper

Springer is part of Springer Science+Business Media (www.springer.com)

This book is dedicated to my wife, Demetria and my staff Barbara, Carrie, Rolanda and Linda. Without their help and support this book would not have transpired.

Preface

Over the past decade presence of chronic kidney disease (CKD) has been increasingly recognized as an independent risk factor for cardiovascular events and death. The incidence of both CKD and heart failure is increasing worldwide and the interaction focusing on the regulatory changes that occur in the physiology of the kidney as a function of a failing heart is not thoroughly discussed in any one place. This book is a compilation of specific chapters from the main textbook, *The Kidney in Heart Failure*. These chapters were selected as key to the understanding of changes in the failing kidney during heart failure. A nephrologist and cardiologist co-authored most chapters so as to present a unified perspective on the respective topics. The book covers specific topics focused on relevance to clinicians managing patients in a broad range of clinical practice settings. It focuses on pathophysiology as well as both pharmacologic and nonpharmacologic management. It places particular focus on common conundrums in heart failure management such as changes in serum creatinine following initiation of renin–angiotensin–aldosterone blockers, edema management in hypoalbuminemic patients, and other such topics. Lastly, whole chapters are dedicated to the use of combination therapy and drug adherence as well as markers of disease, CKD risk and improvement. The reader who reads part or this entire book will be much better versed on the subtleties of management of the cardiorenal patient so as to optimize reduction in cardiovascular mortality and preservation of kidney function.

Chicago, IL, USA   George L. Bakris

Contents

**Chronic Kidney Disease and Heart Failure: Epidemiology
and Outcomes**.. 1
Ruth C. Campbell and Ali Ahmed

**Changes in Kidney Function Following Heart Failure Treatment:
Focus on Renin–Angiotensin System Blockade**... 11
Mohammed Shakaib and George L. Bakris

Hyperkalemia Risk and Treatment of Heart Failure 23
Julian Segura and Luis M. Ruilope

Management of Heart Failure with Renal Artery Ischaemia 43
Andrew K. Roy and Patrick Murray

Combination Therapy in Hypertension Treatment 59
Raymond V. Oliva and George L. Bakris

**Edema Mechanisms in the Heart Failure Patient
and Treatment Options**.. 73
Domenic A. Sica

Ultrafiltration and Heart Failure... 91
Paul Chacko, Donald Kikta Jr., and William T. Abraham

Index.. 113

Contributors

William T. Abraham Ohio State University Medical Center, Columbus, OH, USA

Ali Ahmed Division of Gerontology, Geriatrics and Palliative Care, Department of Medicine, School of Medicine, University of Alabama at Birmingham and VA Medical Center, Birmingham, AL, USA

George L. Bakris ASH Comprehensive Hypertension Center, Department of Medicine University of Chicago Medicine, Chicago, IL, USA

Ruth C. Campbell Division of Nephrology, Department of Medicine, School of Medicine, Medical University of South Carolina, Charleston, SC, USA

Paul Chacko Cardiology Division, Internal Medicine Department, The Ohio State University Medical Center, Columbus, OH, USA

Donald Kikta Jr. Cardiology Division, Internal Medicine Department, The Ohio State University Medical Center, Columbus, OH, USA

Patrick Murray Clinical Pharmacology, University College Dublin, UCD-Mater Clinical Research Centre, Mater Misericordiae University Hospital, Dublin, Ireland

Raymond V. Oliva Section of Hypertension, Department of Medicine, Philippine General Hospital, University of the Philippines College of Medicine, Manila, Philippines

Andrew K. Roy Cardiology Department, Mater Misericordiae University Hospital, Dublin, Ireland

Luis M. Ruilope Hypertension Unit, Nephrology Department, Madrid, Spain

Julian Segura Hypertension Unit, Nephrology Department, Madrid, Spain

Mohammed Shakaib Section of Nephrology, University of Chicago, Pritzker School of Medicine, Chicago, IL, USA

Domenic A. Sica Clinical Pharmacology and Hypertension, Virginia Commonwealth University Health System, Richmond, VA, USA

Chronic Kidney Disease and Heart Failure: Epidemiology and Outcomes

Ruth C. Campbell and Ali Ahmed

Epidemiology of Heart Failure

Heart failure (HF) is a multidisciplinary, complex cardiovascular syndrome with complicated pathophysiology and poor prognosis. Despite advances in treatment, mortality remains high. After the diagnosis of HF, 20% of patients will die within 1 year, and 80% under the age of 65 years will die within 8 years [1]. Over an estimated $37 billion was spent on HF care in 2009. Because over 80% of HF patients are ≥65 years [1], most of these patients suffer from one or more comorbidities. Findings from over 100,000 HF patients in the Acute Decompensated Heart Failure National Registry (ADHERE) suggest that 57% of HF patients have coronary artery disease, 73% have hypertension, 44% have diabetes mellitus, and over 60% have chronic kidney disease (CKD) [2, 3]. CKD is an increasingly recognized marker of poor outcomes in HF. This article will review the epidemiology of both CKD and HF, and the impact of CKD on HF treatment and outcomes.

Epidemiology of CKD

An estimated 13% of the US population ≥20 years of age have CKD, an increase of 10% from 20 years ago [4]. This increase in the prevalence of CKD has been attributed to the increased prevalence of diabetes, hypertension, and obesity during

Originally published in Bakris, The Kidney in Heart Failure, ISBN: 978-1-4614-3693-5

R.C. Campbell (✉)
Division of Nephrology, Department of Medicine, School of Medicine,
Medical University of South Carolina, Charleston, SC, USA
e-mail: campberc@musc.edu

A. Ahmed
Division of Gerontology, Geriatrics and Palliative Care, Department of Medicine, School of
Medicine, University of Alabama at Birmingham and VA Medical Center, Birmingham, AL, USA

G.L. Bakris (ed.), *Managing the Kidney when the Heart is Failing*,
DOI 10.1007/978-1-4614-3691-1_1, © Springer Science+Business Media New York 2012

that period. Age is also an important risk factor [4]. Studies of older populations have demonstrated prevalence rates of 22–43% [5, 6], and CKD is frequently accompanied by other comorbidities such as diabetes, hypertension, and prior cardiovascular disease.

Diagnosis of CKD

The diagnosis of CKD is based on three factors: an estimate of glomerular filtration rate (eGFR), the presence of renal damage (such as proteinuria or hematuria), and chronicity (>3 months) [7]. Serum creatinine alone should not be used to make the diagnosis of CKD as it is not a sensitive marker of GFR [7]. Reduced eGFR <60 ml/min/1.73 m^2 body surface area (BSA) for more than 3 months is sufficient for the diagnosis of CKD. CKD is divided into five stages based on eGFR and other evidence of kidney damage (Table 1) [8].

Estimated GFR is usually calculated by creatinine-based prediction equations because they are less cumbersome and more accurate than timed creatinine clearance studies. The MDRD, Cockcroft-Gault and CKD-EPI equations are widely used (Box 1). The MDRD equation has been validated in whites, African Americans, and patients with diabetes [10]. A limitation of these equations is that they underestimate GFR when GFR is ≥60 ml/min/1.73 m^2 and the newly developed CKD-EPI equation is believed to be more accurate for this population [11]. None of these equations have been specifically validated in HF populations.

All three of these equations are based on creatinine, which makes them less accurate when serum creatinine production is abnormal, such as in severe malnutrition, muscle wasting, limb amputation, or cirrhosis. Aging is also associated with loss of muscle mass, and there has been some debate as to whether the creatinine-based eGFR equations are overly sensitive, particularly in the elderly and women [12]. Cystatin C, a cysteine proteinase inhibitor that is freely filtered at the glomerulus, has been proposed as an alternative to creatinine-based estimates of GFR [13–15]. However, cystatin C is also influenced by factors such as hypothyroidism, tobacco use and inflammation, and is not widely available [16, 17].

Table 1 Stages of chronic kidney disease [8]

Stage	Description	GFR[a] (ml/min/1.73 m^2 of body surface area)
1	Kidney damage[b] with normal or increased GFR	>90
2	Kidney damage with mildly decreased GFR	60–89
3	Moderately decreased GFR	30–59
4	Severely decreased GFR	15–29
5	Kidney failure	<15 or dialysis

Adapted from [9]. With kind permission from Elsevier
[a] GFR estimated from serum creatinine by abbreviated Modification of Diet in Renal Disease Study equation based on age, sex, race, and calibration for serum creatinine
[b] Kidney damage includes proteinuria or albuminuria, hematuria or renal imaging abnormalities

Box 1 Estimates of glomerular filtration rate in adults

Abbreviated (4-variable) MDRD Study Equation:

$$\text{GFR (ml/min/1.73 m}^2) = 175 \times (S_{cr})^{-1.154} \times (\text{Age})^{-0.203} \times (0.742 \text{ if female})$$
$$\times (1.212 \text{ if black})$$

Cockcroft Gault Equation:

$$\text{Creatinine Clearance (ml/min)} = \frac{(140 - \text{age}) \times \text{lean body weight (kg)}}{\text{Serum creatinine (mg/dl)} \times 72} \times 0.85 \text{ if female}$$

CKD-EPI Equation:

$$\text{GFR (ml/min/1.73 m}^2) = 141 \times \min (S_{cr}/\kappa, 1)\alpha \times \max(S_{cr}/\kappa, 1) - 1.209 \times 0.993$$
$$\text{Age} \times 1.018 \text{ [if female]} \times 1.159 \text{ [if black]}$$

where S_{cr} is serum creatinine in mg/dL, κ is 0.7 for females and 0.9 for males, α is −0.329 for females and −0.411 for males, min indicates the minimum of S_{cr}/κ or 1, and max indicates the maximum of S_{cr}/κ or 1.

While eGFR is an important component of the CKD classification system, the presence of proteinuria is a very strong predictor of both the risk of ESRD and cardiovascular events and should not be overlooked [18–20]. Proteinuria found on dipstick testing should always be quantified with a urinary albumin or protein to creatinine ratio from a random urine sample, or a timed urine collection.

Epidemiology of CKD in HF

Patients with high serum creatinine levels have often been excluded from randomized clinical trials in HF. Data from these trials are therefore not suitable for the estimation of CKD in HF [21–23]. In contrast, data from HF registries, which do not routinely exclude these patients, are more suitable for the estimation of the prevalence of CKD. Findings from major HF registries suggest that nearly 60% of HF patients have CKD (Table 2) [9].

Risk Factors for CKD in HF

Prospective epidemiological data on the risk of CKD in patients with HF are scarce. Findings from cross-sectional studies suggest that age, baseline GFR, diabetes, hypertension, body mass index, smoking, ethnicity, education, and cardiovascular

Table 2 Prevalence of chronic kidney disease in heart failure (HF)

Study	Data source	Number of HF patients	Mean age	Women (%)	African American (%)	Method to define CKD	Prevalence of CKD (%)
HF registries							
Heywood et al. [3]	ADHERE	118,465	72	52	21	MDRD	64
Masoudi et al. [24]	NHCP	62,376	79	58	10	MDRD	67
RCT of HF							
Hillege et al. [22]	CHARM	2,680	65	33	4	MDRD	36
Khan et al. [23]	SOLVD	6,440	60	14	12	MDRD	33
Ahmed et al. [21]	DIG	7,788	64	25	15	MDRD	45
Population studies of HF							
Ahmed A	CHS	262	75	52	20	MDRD	53
Ahmed A	FHS	70	74	70	0	MDRD	74

Adapted from [9]. With kind permission from Elsevier

CHS Cardiovascular Health Study, *FHS* Framingham Heart Study, *MDRD* Modification of Diet in Renal Disease

disease are associated with CKD [25]. Because of the high prevalence of many of these risk factors in HF patients, the risk of CKD in HF is also likely high. Findings from the ADHERE registry suggest that age, sex, race, and hypertension are associated with CKD [3]. In that study, the proportion of African Americans among HF patients with stages 3 and 4 CKD was 15% and 15%, respectively. However, among those with stage 5 CKD (kidney failure), 33% were African Americans, suggesting a higher prevalence of more advanced CKD among African Americans [3]. A similar association between race and CKD was also observed in REasons for Geographic and Racial Differences in Stroke (REGARDS), a study of stroke risk in community-dwelling adults ≥45 years of age [5].

Findings from the ADHERE registry also suggest that the prevalence of diabetes was higher among those with higher stages of CKD [3]. The prevalences of coronary artery disease and systolic HF (ejection fraction <40%), on the other hand, were low among those with stage 5 CKD [3]. This may in part be due to the higher mortality associated with coronary artery disease or low ejection fraction among HF patients with stage 5 CKD [26, 27]. Similar associations with these risk factors are also observed in ambulatory chronic HF patients [21, 22].

CKD as a Risk Factor for HF

Because HF and CKD share common risk factors that often co-exist, it may be difficult to determine whether CKD in HF is a cause of prevalent or incident CKD, or a manifestation of cardiorenal syndrome [28–30]. Data from the Cardiovascular Health Study indicate that among older adults, increasing baseline serum creatinine levels were associated with a graded increase in the risk for incident HF [31]. However, it is unknown whether CKD as defined by eGFR <60 ml/min/1.73 m^2 BSA would also predict incident HF in that study. A further analysis of the Cardiovascular Health Study suggests that among older adults without baseline CKD, pre-clinical CKD as identified by cystatin C was associated with increased risk of HF [13].

Prognostic Implications of CKD in HF

The presence of CKD is associated with poor prognosis in HF and CKD can be used to risk-stratify HF patients for targeted intervention [3, 21, 22, 32–35]. The risk of death increases as GFR decreases and may be more strongly associated with a reduced GFR than with a reduced left ventricular ejection fraction [28]. In one study, the effect of CKD has been shown to be more pronounced in ambulatory patients with diastolic HF than in those with systolic HF (Fig. 1) [21].

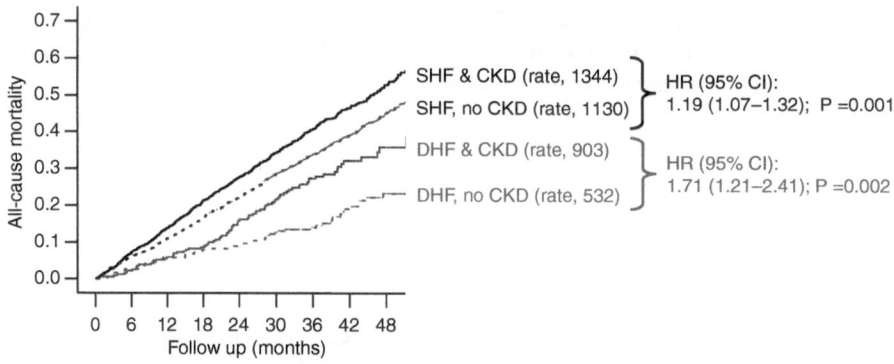

Fig. 1 Kaplan–Meier plots for cumulative risk of chronic kidney disease (CKD)-associated all-cause death in patients with systolic heart failure (SHF) and diastolic heart failure (DHF), with rates of death (expressed per 10,000 person-years of follow up), and hazard ratio (HR) and 95% confidence interval (CI), when CKD is compared with no CKD. Adapted from [21]. With kind permission from Elsevier

Therapeutic Implications of CKD in Heart Failure

There are two aspects in the therapeutic implications of CKD in HF: (1) the impact of the presence of CKD on the receipt of evidence-based therapy, and (2) the importance of administration of such therapy to HF patients with CKD. Angiotensin-converting enzyme (ACE) inhibitors and angiotensin receptor blockers (ARBs) have been shown to reduce mortality in patients with systolic HF [36]. However, these drugs are often underused in HF patients with CKD. One of the reasons for this underuse is the perception that the increase in serum creatinine associated with the use of these drugs may be an indication of worsening kidney function [37, 38]. This is despite the fact that the anticipated rise in serum creatinine associated with the use of ACEi inhibitors and ARBs is often mild (<30%) and reversible, and is considered a marker of their effectiveness [39]. ACE inhibitors and ARBs have been shown to reduce the progression of kidney damage in a wide spectrum of patients with kidney disease, particularly those with proteinuria [40]. Therefore, these drugs may be both cardio- and reno-protective in systolic HF patients with CKD [41, 42].

Although patients with CKD were often excluded from most randomized clinical trials of ACE inhibitors and ARBs in HF, post hoc and subgroup analyses and other observational data suggest that these drugs may also be effective in HF patients with CKD, and the absolute benefit may even be greater in patients with CKD than in those without CKD [24, 35, 37, 43, 44]. The cardio-protective benefit of ACE inhibitors and ARBs is not well established in diastolic HF. These patients may benefit from the renoprotective effects of these drugs, which may indirectly improve prognosis [44], although this has not been demonstrated in large-scale randomized clinical trials.

Summary

HF is common and has a poor prognosis. CKD is common in HF and the presence of CKD further worsens the prognosis of HF. The presence of CKD is a marker of poor prognosis, regardless of ejection fraction, and these patients should be appropriately treated with inhibitors of the renin–angiotensin system. Any associated hypertension, diabetes, or other shared risk factors should also be appropriately treated. Clinicians should routinely risk-stratify HF patients by the presence of CKD and take preventive and therapeutic measures based on current guidelines and appropriate nephrology consultation.

Acknowledgments Dr. Campbell is supported by the National Institutes of Health through a grant from the National Institute of Diabetes and Digestive and Kidney Diseases, 1-K23-DK-64649. Dr. Ahmed is supported by the National Institutes of Health through grants (R01-HL085561, R01-HL085561-S and R01-HL097047) from the National Heart, Lung, and Blood Institute and a generous gift from Ms. Jean B. Morris of Birmingham, Alabama.

References

1. Lloyd-Jones D, Adams RJ, Brown TM, et al. Heart disease and stroke statistics—2010 update: a report from the American Heart Association. Circulation. 2010;121:e46–215.
2. Adams Jr KF, Fonarow GC, Emerman CL, et al. Characteristics and outcomes of patients hospitalized for heart failure in the United States: rationale, design, and preliminary observations from the first 100,000 cases in the Acute Decompensated Heart Failure National Registry (ADHERE). Am Heart J. 2005;149:209–16.
3. Heywood JT, Fonarow GC, Costanzo MR, Mathur VS, Wigneswaran JR, Wynne J. High prevalence of renal dysfunction and its impact on outcome in 118,465 patients hospitalized with acute decompensated heart failure: a report from the ADHERE database. J Card Fail. 2007; 13:422–30.
4. Coresh J, Selvin E, Stevens LA, et al. Prevalence of chronic kidney disease in the United States. JAMA. 2007;298:2038–47.
5. McClellan W, Warnock DG, McClure L, et al. Racial differences in the prevalence of chronic kidney disease among participants in the Reasons for Geographic and Racial Differences in Stroke (REGARDS) Cohort Study. J Am Soc Nephrol. 2006;17:1710–5.
6. Shlipak MG, Fried LF, Cushman M, et al. Cardiovascular mortality risk in chronic kidney disease: comparison of traditional and novel risk factors. JAMA. 2005;293:1737–45.
7. Stevens LA, Coresh J, Feldman HI, et al. Evaluation of the modification of diet in renal disease study equation in a large diverse population. J Am Soc Nephrol. 2007;18:2749–57.
8. The National Kidney Foundation. K/DOQI clinical practice guidelines for chronic kidney disease: evaluation, classification, and stratification. Am J Kidney Dis. 2002;39:S1–266.
9. Ahmed A, Campbell RC. Epidemiology of chronic kidney disease in heart failure. Heart Fail Clin. 2008;4:387–99.
10. Stevens LA, Coresh J, Greene T, Levey AS. Assessing kidney function—measured and estimated glomerular filtration rate. N Engl J Med. 2006;354:2473–83.
11. Levey AS, Stevens LA, Schmid CH, et al. A new equation to estimate glomerular filtration rate. Ann Intern Med. 2009;150:604–12.

12. Glassock RJ, Winearls C. CKD in the elderly. Am J Kidney Dis. 2008;52:803 [author reply 803–4].

13. Shlipak MG, Katz R, Sarnak MJ, et al. Cystatin C and prognosis for cardiovascular and kidney outcomes in elderly persons without chronic kidney disease. Ann Intern Med. 2006;145: 237–46.

14. Randers E, Erlandsen EJ, Pedersen OL, Hasling C, Danielsen H. Serum cystatin C as an endogenous parameter of the renal function in patients with normal to moderately impaired kidney function. Clin Nephrol. 2000;54:203–9.

15. Hojs R, Bevc S, Ekart R, Gorenjak M, Puklavec L. Serum cystatin C as an endogenous marker of renal function in patients with mild to moderate impairment of kidney function. Nephrol Dial Transplant. 2006;21:1855–62.

16. Herget-Rosenthal S, Bokenkamp A, Hofmann W. How to estimate GFR-serum creatinine, serum cystatin C or equations? Clin Biochem. 2007;40:153–61.

17. Knight EL, Verhave JC, Spiegelman D, et al. Factors influencing serum cystatin C levels other than renal function and the impact on renal function measurement. Kidney Int. 2004;65: 1416–21.

18. de Zeeuw D, Remuzzi G, Parving HH, et al. Albuminuria, a therapeutic target for cardiovascular protection in type 2 diabetic patients with nephropathy. Circulation. 2004;110:921–7.

19. Ibsen H, Olsen MH, Wachtell K, et al. Reduction in albuminuria translates to reduction in cardiovascular events in hypertensive patients: losartan intervention for endpoint reduction in hypertension study. Hypertension. 2005;45:198–202.

20. Ruggenenti P, Perna A, Mosconi L, Pisoni R, Remuzzi G. Urinary protein excretion rate is the best independent predictor of ESRF in non-diabetic proteinuric chronic nephropathies. "Gruppo Italiano di Studi Epidemiologici in Nefrologia" (GISEN). Kidney Int. 1998;53:1209–16.

21. Ahmed A, Rich MW, Sanders PW, et al. Chronic kidney disease associated mortality in diastolic versus systolic heart failure: a propensity matched study. Am J Cardiol. 2007;99:393–8.

22. Hillege HL, Nitsch D, Pfeffer MA, et al. Renal function as a predictor of outcome in a broad spectrum of patients with heart failure. Circulation. 2006;113:671–8.

23. Khan NA, Ma I, Thompson CR, et al. Kidney function and mortality among patients with left ventricular systolic dysfunction. J Am Soc Nephrol. 2006;17:244–53.

24. Masoudi FA, Baillie CA, Wang Y, et al. The complexity and cost of drug regimens of older patients hospitalized with heart failure in the United States, 1998–2001. Arch Intern Med. 2005;165:2069–76.

25. Fox CS, Larson MG, Leip EP, Culleton B, Wilson PW, Levy D. Predictors of new-onset kidney disease in a community-based population. JAMA. 2004;291:844–50.

26. Goodman WG, Goldin J, Kuizon BD, et al. Coronary-artery calcification in young adults with end-stage renal disease who are undergoing dialysis. N Engl J Med. 2000;342:1478–83.

27. Herzog CA, Ma JZ, Collins AJ. Comparative survival of dialysis patients in the United States after coronary angioplasty, coronary artery stenting, and coronary artery bypass surgery and impact of diabetes. Circulation. 2002;106:2207–11.

28. Bongartz LG, Cramer MJ, Doevendans PA, Joles JA, Braam B. The severe cardiorenal syndrome: 'Guyton revisited'. Eur Heart J. 2005;26:11–7.

29. Schrier RW. Cardiorenal versus renocardiac syndrome: is there a difference? Nat Clin Pract Nephrol. 2007;3:637.

30. Shlipak MG, Massie BM. The clinical challenge of cardiorenal syndrome. Circulation. 2004;110:1514–7.

31. Gottdiener JS, Arnold AM, Aurigemma GP, et al. Predictors of congestive heart failure in the elderly: the Cardiovascular Health Study. J Am Coll Cardiol. 2000;35:1628–37.

32. Campbell RC, Sui X, Filippatos G, et al. Association of chronic kidney disease with outcomes in chronic heart failure: a propensity-matched study. Nephrol Dial Transplant. 2009;24:186–93.

33. Cowie MR, Komajda M, Murray-Thomas T, Underwood J, Ticho B. Prevalence and impact of worsening renal function in patients hospitalized with decompensated heart failure: results of the prospective outcomes study in heart failure (POSH). Eur Heart J. 2006;27:1216–22.

34. Damman K, Navis G, Voors AA, et al. Worsening renal function and prognosis in heart failure: systematic review and meta-analysis. J Card Fail. 2007;13:599–608.
35. Ezekowitz J, McAlister FA, Humphries KH, et al. The association among renal insufficiency, pharmacotherapy, and outcomes in 6,427 patients with heart failure and coronary artery disease. J Am Coll Cardiol. 2004;44:1587–92.
36. Hunt SA, Abraham WT, Chin MH, et al. ACC/AHA 2005 Guideline Update for the Diagnosis and Management of Chronic Heart Failure in the Adult. A report of the American College of Cardiology/American Heart Association Task Force on Practice Guidelines (Writing Committee to Update the 2001 Guidelines for the Evaluation and Management of Heart Failure). Developed in collaboration with the American College of Chest Physicians and the International Society for Heart and Lung Transplantation. Endorsed by the Heart Rhythm Society. Circulation. 2005;112:e154–235.
37. Ahmed A, Kiefe CI, Allman RM, Sims RV, DeLong JF. Survival benefits of angiotensin-converting enzyme inhibitors in older heart failure patients with perceived contraindications. J Am Geriatr Soc. 2002;50:1659–66.
38. Masoudi FA, Rathore SS, Wang Y, et al. National patterns of use and effectiveness of angiotensin-converting enzyme inhibitors in older patients with heart failure and left ventricular systolic dysfunction. Circulation. 2004;110:724–31.
39. Bakris GL, Weir MR. Angiotensin-converting enzyme inhibitor-associated elevations in serum creatinine: is this a cause for concern? Arch Intern Med. 2000;160:685–93.
40. Maschio G, Alberti D, Janin G, et al. Effect of the angiotensin-converting-enzyme inhibitor benazepril on the progression of chronic renal insufficiency. The Angiotensin-Converting-Enzyme Inhibition in Progressive Renal Insufficiency Study Group. N Engl J Med. 1996; 334:939–45.
41. Ahmed A, Love TE, Sui X, Rich MW. Effects of angiotensin-converting enzyme inhibitors in systolic heart failure patients with chronic kidney disease: a propensity score analysis. J Card Fail. 2006;12:499–506.
42. Berger AK, Duval S, Manske C, et al. Angiotensin-converting enzyme inhibitors and angiotensin receptor blockers in patients with congestive heart failure and chronic kidney disease. Am Heart J. 2007;153:1064–73.
43. McAlister FA, Ezekowitz J, Tonelli M, Armstrong PW. Renal insufficiency and heart failure: prognostic and therapeutic implications from a prospective cohort study. Circulation. 2004; 109:1004–9.
44. Ahmed A, Allman RM, Aban I, et al. Renin-angiotensin system inhibition and reduction in all-cause mortality in hospitalized elderly diastolic heart failure patients with chronic kidney disease: a propensity-matched study. Eur Heart J. 2009;30:866.

Changes in Kidney Function Following Heart Failure Treatment: Focus on Renin–Angiotensin System Blockade

Mohammed Shakaib and George L. Bakris

Introduction

Given that the increased activation of the renin–angiotensin system (RAS) results in adverse cardiovascular hemodynamics and remodeling effects, it therefore follows (and is, of course, well proven in a plethora of trials) that therapies which block RAS, namely angiotensin-converting enzyme inhibitors (ACEI), angiotensin receptor blockers (ARBs), and aldosterone antagonists, are beneficial in this setting.

The clinical management of HF patients with acute or chronic kidney disease is complex. While on the one hand, these patients have a poor prognosis and thus stand to greatly benefit from the therapies that reduce mortality and improve quality of life, these patients are often vulnerable to feared side effects such as worsening renal failure or hyperkalemia.

Treatment of Heart Failure

Heart Failure: A Clinical Syndrome

The 2005 ACC/AHA Guideline for the Diagnosis and Management of Chronic Heart Failure in the Adult defines HF as a complex syndrome that can result from

Originally published in Bakris, The Kidney in Heart Failure, ISBN: 978-1-4614-3693-5

M. Shakaib
Section of Nephrology, University of Chicago, Pritzker School of Medicine, Chicago, IL, USA

G.L. Bakris (✉)
ASH Comprehensive Hypertension Center, Department of Medicine, University of Chicago Medicine, 5841 S. Maryland Avenue, MC1027, Chicago, IL 60637, USA
e-mail: gbakris@gmail.com

G.L. Bakris (ed.), *Managing the Kidney when the Heart is Failing*,   11
DOI 10.1007/978-1-4614-3691-1_2, © Springer Science+Business Media New York 2012

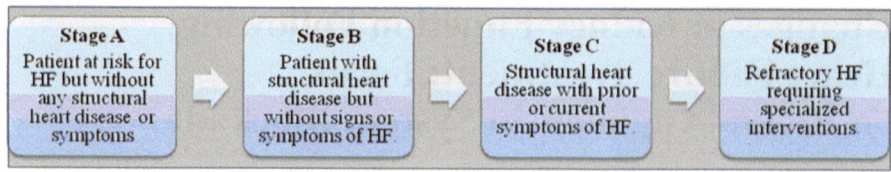

Fig. 1 Stages of heart failure

any structural or functional cardiac disorder that impairs the ability of the ventricle to fill with or eject blood.

The development of HF can be categorized into four stages (Fig. 1):

- Stage A—Patient at risk for HF but without any structural heart disease or symptoms.
- Stage B—Patient with structural heart disease but without signs or symptoms of HF.
- Stage C—Structural heart disease with prior or current symptoms of HF.
- Stage D—Refractory HF requiring specialized interventions.

Benefits of Therapies Blocking RAS: Clinical Studies

Benefits of ACE Inhibitors

ACE inhibitors were initially developed for use as vasodilators, but when their clinical benefits proved to be out of proportion to that expected, it was recognized that there were mechanisms other than their vasodilatory properties, which accounted for this success. Figure 2 shows the pathway for angiotensin-II formation as well as the site of action of ACEI, ARB, and aldosterone blockers. While human studies have demonstrated that over 80% of the generation of angiotensin-II is by the ACE pathway, there is also a contribution from the chymase pathway, a protease which is found in interstitial cells [1].

ACE inhibitors have demonstrated a significant reduction in mortality of patients with HF in multiple, large, prospective, randomized trials [2–4]. Overall, there is a significant reduction in death, MI, and hospital admission for HF.

Benefits of ARBs

ARBs block the angiotensin-II type I receptors (Fig. 2) and thus, act irrespective of how the angiotensin-II is generated. Unlike ACEI, they have no influence on bradykinin and thus have the advantage of eliminating the cough, which sometimes results from therapy with ACEI. ARBs seem to exert renal and cardiac hemodynamic effects similar to ACE inhibitors. Clinically, they have shown to be reasonable alternatives to ACEI as they have demonstrated efficacy in multiple randomized trials [5–7].

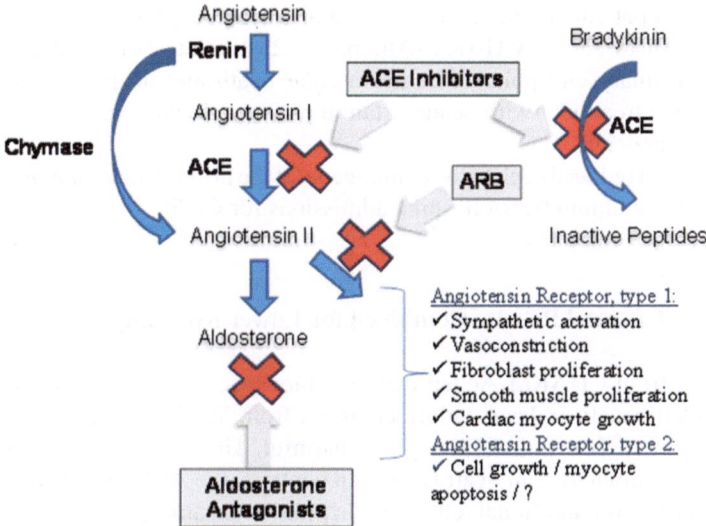

Fig. 2 Renin–angiotensin–aldosterone system and its inhibitors

The Evaluation of Losartan in the Elderly (ELITE I) [8] was the first long-term clinical trial which compared an ACEI (captopril) to an ARB (losartan) in patients with heart failure and reduced left ventricular ejection fraction. Surprisingly, this trial demonstrated decrease in all-cause mortality in patients treated with Losartan. Losartan was generally better tolerated than captopril (12.2% discontinued treatment with losartan vs. 21% with captopril, $p=0.002$), although the frequency of persisting increases in serum creatinine was the same in both groups (10.5%).

In order to confirm whether losartan conferred a survival advantage, the large ELITE II [9] study was conducted. There was no statistically significant difference in all-cause mortality (11.7% vs. 10.4%), sudden death, or resuscitated arrests between the two treatment groups although, again, fewer patients treated with the ARB had to discontinue therapy due to adverse events.

In the evaluation of strategies for left ventricular dysfunction (RESOLVD) pilot study [10], candesartan alone was as effective, safe, and tolerable as enalapril. The combination of candesartan and enalapril was more beneficial for preventing left ventricular remodeling than either candesartan or enalapril alone suggesting that there might be an advantage to combination therapy with both ACEI and ARB.

In the Valsartan Heart Failure Trial (Val-HeFT) [11], when added to prescribed therapy, valsartan significantly reduced the combined end point of mortality and morbidity by 13.2%. However, the post hoc showed an adverse effect on mortality and morbidity in the subgroup receiving valsartan, an ACE inhibitor, and a beta-blocker, thus raising concern about the potential safety of using combination therapy.

The CHARM trial represented one of the largest trials to ever be conducted in HF patients [12–14]. The three parallel arms of this study yielded the following conclusions: (1) ARBs reduce morbidity and mortality in HF patients; (2) ARBs can be used safely in patients intolerant of ACEI and, when used in this setting, provide a similar benefit to ACEI (CHARM-Alternative 23% relative-risk reduction in the composite primary end point of cardiovascular death and hospital admission for CHF); and (3) treatment with candesartan in patients already on ACEI and a beta-blocker is beneficial.

Candesartan reduced each of the components of the primary outcome significantly, as well as the total number of hospital admissions for CHF.

"Should ACEI and ARBs Be Combined for Lower Mortality"

The finding from CHARM-Added that dual blockade of the RAS system trended toward added benefit in heart failure contrasts from Val-HeFT that suggested that addition of an ARB to an ACEI might be harmful. Thus, there are no solid data to support this combination in heart failure. In contrast, the ACEI and ARB combination is beneficial for additional reductions in proteinuria among those with advanced proteinuric kidney disease. A recent comprehensive meta-analysis by Kunz et al. [15] concluded that while reduction in proteinuria is similar between ACEI and ARBs, their combination is more effective than either drug alone. The applicability of these results is limited as reduction in proteinuria is only a marker for slowing of kidney disease progression and cannot be extrapolated to earlier stage nephropathy that involves better kidney function and normo- or micro-albuminuria.

The adverse effects of combination ACEI and ARBs in patients with symptomatic left ventricular dysfunction were examined in a review by Phillips et al. [16]. In four studies representing 17,337 patients, the combination of ACEI plus ARB vs. ACEI was associated with significant increases in medication discontinuations because of adverse effects in patients with chronic heart failure

Heart Failure Therapy: Aldosterone Antagonists

Spironolactone (aldactone) acts by direct competition with aldosterone for binding to the mineralocorticoid receptor. It thus reduces the avidity of the distal nephron for sodium reabsorption and results in sodium excretion. While spironolactone therapy substantially reduces the likelihood of hypokalemia from diuretic therapy, it also increases the risk of hyperkalemia [17], especially in patients with renal insufficiency or when used concurrently with ACE inhibitors. However, a recent analysis of the *Eplerenone Post-Acute Myocardial Infarction Heart Failure Efficacy and Survival Study* (EPHESUS) demonstrated that there was a benefit on cardiovascular mortality in people with kidney disease up to a serum potassium of 5.7 mEq/L [18].

The observation that aldosterone may be secreted independently of angiotensin-II suggested that direct blockade of aldosterone may have an important role in the treatment of heart failure. The *Randomized Aldactone Evaluation Study Investigators*

Table 1 ACC/AHA indications for ACEI and ARBs and heart failure stage

Heart failure stage	Use of ACE inhibitors	Use of ARB
A	All patients with history of: (class IIa) Atherosclerotic vascular disease Diabetes mellitus Hypertension with cardiovascular risk factors	
B	All patients post MI (class I) All patients with reduced EF and no symptoms (class I)	All patients post MI without HF who are intolerant of ACEI (class I) All patients with reduced EF and no symptoms who are intolerant of ACEI (class IIa)
C	All patients with current or prior symptoms of HF and reduced LVEF (class I) (*Note*: Routine combined use of ACEI, ARB, and aldosterone antagonist is not recommended—class III)	All patients with current or prior symptoms of HF and reduced LVEF who are intolerant of ACEI (class I) ARB use as first-line therapy (alternative to ACEI) for patients with mild-to-moderate HF and reduced LVEF (class IIa) Addition of ARB in persistently symptomatic patients with reduced EF who are already being treated with conventional therapy (class IIb)

Recommendation class: class I—conditions for which there is evidence and/or general agreement that a given procedure or treatment is beneficial, useful, and effective; class II—conditions for which there is conflicting evidence and/or a divergence of opinion about the usefulness/efficacy of a procedure or treatment; class IIa—weight of evidence/opinion is in favor of usefulness/efficacy; class IIb—usefulness/efficacy is less well established by evidence/opinion; class III—conditions for which there is evidence and/or general agreement that a procedure/treatment is not useful/ effective and is some cases may be harmful

(RALES) [19] study in patients with severe (EF < 35%), NYHA classes III–IV heart failure showed a 30% reduction in the risk of death among patients in the spironolactone group.

The EPHESUS randomized 6,632 patient on optimal baseline medical therapy (i.e., 75% were on beta-blocker therapy, and 86% were on ACEI or ARBs) to eplerenone or placebo [20]. The rate of the primary end point, death from cardiovascular causes or hospitalization for cardiovascular events, was reduced by 13% in eplerenone group, but there is a need to monitor for hyperkalemia and adjust dose accordingly.

Use of ACEI Vs. ARBs in Heart Failure: What Do the Guidelines Tell Us?

Table 1 lists the indications for ACEI and ARB for each class of HF as well as the ACC/AHA designated recommendation class (class I—conditions for which there is evidence and/or general agreement that a given procedure or treatment is beneficial, useful, and effective; class II—conditions for which there is conflicting evidence and/or a divergence of opinion about the usefulness/efficacy of a procedure or treatment; class IIa—weight of evidence/opinion is in favor of usefulness/efficacy;

Table 2 RAS inhibitors used in treatment of various stages of heart failure

Drug	Stage A	Stage B	Stage C
ACE inhibitors			
Benazepril	H	–	–
Captopril	H, DN	Post MI	HF
Enalapril	H, DN	Asympt LVSD	HF
Fosinopril	H	–	HF
Lisinopril	H, DN	Post MI	HF
Moexipril	H	–	–
Perindopril	H, CV Risk	–	–
Quinapril	H	–	HF
Ramipril	H, CV Risk	Post MI	Post MI
Trandolapril	H	Post MI	Post MI
Angiotensin receptor blockers			
Candesartan	H	–	HF
Eprosartan	H	–	–
Irbesartan	H, DN	–	–
Losartan	H, DN	CV Risk	–
Olmesartan	H	–	–
Telmisartan	H	–	–
Valsartan	H	DN post MI	Post MI, HF
Aldosterone blockers			
Eplerenone	H	Post MI	Post MI
Spironolactone	H	–	HF

Asympt LVSD indicates asymptomatic left ventricular systolic dysfunction, *CV Risk* reduction in future cardiovascular events, *DN* diabetic nephropathy, *H* hypertension, *HF* heart failure, *Post MI*, reduction in heart failure or other cardiac events following myocardial infarction
Adapted from ACC/AHA 2005 Heart Failure Practice Guidelines

class IIb—usefulness/efficacy is less well established by evidence/opinion; class III—conditions for which there is evidence and/or general agreement that a procedure/ treatment is note useful/effective and is some cases may be harmful).

The addition of an aldosterone antagonist is recommended in selected patients with moderately severe to severe symptoms of HF and reduced EF, who can be carefully monitored for preserved renal function and normal potassium concentration. Creatinine should be ≤2.5 mg/dL in men and ≤2.0 mg/dL in women and potassium should be less than 5.0 mEq/L.

Table 2 lists the RAS inhibitors used in the treatment of various stages of heart failure. It is noteworthy that there are different compelling indications for different agents of the same class. This is because these recommendations are based on clinical data that have demonstrated efficacy of a specific agent in a particular subgroup of patients. For instance, while any ACEI and ARB medications can be given to patients with stage A disease that have hypertension, the agents which have demonstrated to be beneficial in patients with diabetic nephropathy are Captopril, Enalapril, Lisinopril, Irbesartan, Losartan, and Valsartan. Similarly, the agents which have shown the most efficacy for patients with stage C heart failure include Captopril, Enalapril, Fosinopril, Lisinopril, Quinapril, Candesartan, Valsartan, and Spironolactone.

Benefits of Heart Failure Therapies: The Real World

Despite the documented benefits of ACE inhibition in treating congestive heart failure, they are underprescribed in many patients who are candidates for their use. Moreover, the dosages used, when prescribed, in many cases are far below those shown to be efficacious for reducing mortality in clinical trials [21].

Given the proven mortality benefit of treatment with ACE inhibitors, ARBs and beta blockers, it is important to ensure that patients who are at higher risk of death receive these therapies. Recognizing the importance of these treatments in reducing morbidity and mortality, the Joint Commission on Accreditation of Health Care Organizations (JCAHO) in collaboration with Centers for Medicare and Medicaid Services (CMS) as well as the American Heart Association (AHA) and American College of Cardiology (ACC) have identified treatment with ACEI and ARB as one of the core measures of quality for patients discharged from the hospital with heart failure.

Indeed, a frequent reason for not using ACEI in patients with HF is the concern for complications attributable to worsened kidney function. Given that among patients with HF, an estimated glomerular filtration rate of <60 mL/min is an independent risk factor associated with poor prognosis [22], it would seem that if anything, these are the patients who would stand to benefit the most from such therapies. Moreover, a rise in creatinine of 30–35% above baseline is associated with better long-term renal outcomes [23]. ACE inhibitors have been studied in HF patients with creatinine levels as high as 3.4 mg/dL. In the CONSENSUS trial, treatment with low-dose Enalapril (2.5 mg) was associated with a relative reduction in mortality of 27% which was attributed, for the most part, to a reduction in death from the progression of heart failure. In CHARM, patients with creatinine of up to 3.0 derived benefit from administration of Candesartan with a benefit, which was irrespective of the degree of underlying renal dysfunction.

Renal Function Following Administration of ACEI and ARB

Kidney Function and Hemodynamics with Heart Failure Pharmacotherapy

Table 3 summarizes the renal hemodynamic effects resulting from activation of various neurohumoral systems as well as the effects that would be expected to occur from therapeutic pharmacologic interventions aimed at blocking these systems. While sympathetic system activation and increase of angiotensin-II cause efferent arteriole constriction, decreased renal blood flow, and proximal sodium reabsorption, blocking these responses with RAS inhibitors would result in decreased efferent arteriole constriction, increased renal blood flow, and decreased water and sodium absorption. These mechanisms are further illustrated in Fig. 3.

Table 3 Effects of activated neurohumoral systems and their blockade on renal hemodynamics in heart failure

	Sympathetic Nerves	ANG II	Aldosterone	ANP	AVP	Diuretics[a]	Alpha-blockers	ACE-I	ARB	Spironolactone	V2-antagonist
Renal blood flow	↓	↓		↑		↑	↑	↑	↑		
Efferent arteriole constriction	↑	↑			↑			↓	↓		
Prox sodium reabsorption	↑	↑		↓				↓	↓		
Distal sodium absorption			↑	↓	↑	↓		↓	↓	↓	
Water absorption				↓	↑	↓					↓
Renin release	↑	↓		↓		↑		↑	↑	↑	
Aldosterone release		↑		↓		↑		↓	↓	↓	

[a]This section refers only to loop diuretics. Moreover, if volume depletion occurs with diuretics, then renal blood flow is reduced with these agents and an indirect increase in efferent arteriolar tone is observed

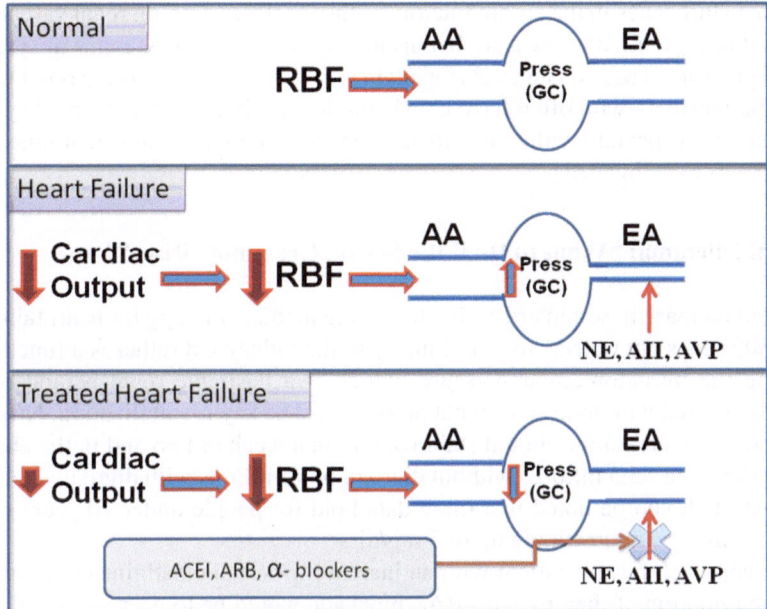

Fig. 3 The impact of neurohormones on the glomerulus: normal, heart failure, and treated heart failure. *AA* afferent arteriole, *EA* efferent arteriole, *RBF* renal blood flow, *GC* glomerular capillary, *NE* norepinephrine, *AII* angiotensin-II, *AVP* arginine vasopressin

Renal Function Worsening Following RAS Blockade

A rise in serum creatinine occurs in about 10–11% of patients with significant heart failure (EF of <20%) treated with ACE inhibitors or ARBs. The mechanisms for this rise in creatinine (reflect an acute fall in glomerular filtration rate) include: (1) loss of angiotensin-II effect on the efferent arteriole leading to a fall in filtration pressure within the glomerulus and (2) significant reduction of blood pressure usually in the presence of intravascular volume depletion, secondary to previous loop diuretic use leading to fall in renal perfusion (Fig. 3).

Studies of left ventricular dysfunction (SOLVD) demonstrated that patients assigned to enalapril had a 33% greater likelihood of decreased renal function than controls. By multivariate analysis, in both the placebo and enalapril groups older age, diuretic therapy, and diabetes were associated with decreased renal function, whereas beta-blocker therapy and higher ejection fraction were renoprotective [24]. It should be noted that the magnitude of renal dysfunction seen with either an ACE inhibitor or ARB is directly proportional to the level of cardiac dysfunction. Hence, the lower the ejection fraction the greater the initial increase in serum creatinine. However, as cardiac function improves serum creatinine will start to fall.

An increase in serum creatinine following improved blood pressure control also occurs in patients with chronic renal failure. In these patients, loss of renal mass leads to disturbances in the autoregulatory ability of the remaining renal vasculature such that intraglomerular pressure begins to vary directly with changes in systemic arterial pressure. These changes also explain why patients with chronic renal failure and hypertension—who often have coexisting heart failure with preserved systolic function—are especially vulnerable to develop an increase in serum creatinine when blood pressure is lowered.

Clinical Dilemma: "What to Do if the Serum Creatinine Rises?"

A limited increase in serum creatinine following medical therapy for heart failure of about 30% does not reflect structural injury to the kidney but rather is a function of lowering the intraglomerular pressure, which is a desirable renal hemodynamic effect associated with long-term renal protection. The key is stabilization. Note that this increase in creatinine should stabilize within a week or two and in the absence of hyperkalemia >5.5 mEq/L, without digoxin or >5 mEq/L with digoxin should be tolerated. It should be noted that these data hold for people under 70 years of age with baseline serum creatinine up to 3 mg/dL.

One approach for the patient with an increase in serum creatinine concentration after the initiation of therapy with RAS blockade would be to decrease the dose of other antihypertensive medications if systolic blood pressure has fallen below 90 mmHg. While this will result in an increase in blood pressure and subsequent return of serum creatinine toward baseline, it is important to emphasize that such an approach prevents maximization of medical therapy shown to have greater risk reduction and thus, is discouraged [23]. In particular, discontinuation of ACEI or ARBs in this scenario would deprive many patients of the proven cardiovascular benefits afforded by these agents. Given this, clinicians who observe a small elevation in creatinine following administration of ACEI or ARBs are advised to continue use of these agents while monitoring the creatinine levels. For most patients, renal function will improve when cardiac function improves; however, even in those whose renal function remains reduced, the long-term renal outcomes will be improved as a result of better blood pressure control [23].

Figure 4 illustrates a recommended approach for initiation of RAS blockade in patient vulnerable to renal insufficiency. This recommendation emphasizes continuation of RAS blockade in patients who have a mild (<30%) increase in creatinine, which eventually stabilizes. This concept is based on the strong association which has been demonstrated between acute increases in serum creatinine of up to 30% that stabilize within the first 2 months of ACEI therapy and long-term preservation of renal function [23].

Hyperkalemia Following RAS Blockade

In addition, ACE inhibitor therapy may cause hyperkalemia in some patients with heart failure, particularly those with baseline glomerular filtration rates of <50% prior to initiation of ACE therapy. Hyperkalemia may be due to reduction in GFR

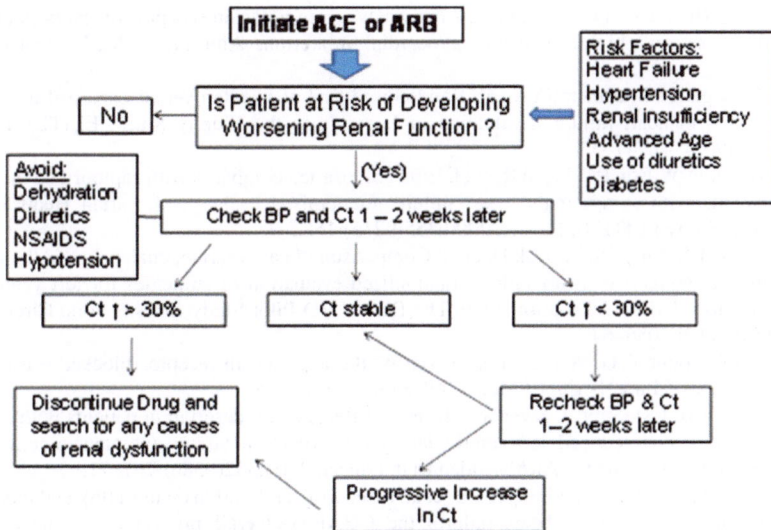

Fig. 4 Approach for initiation of RAS blockade in patient vulnerable to renal insufficiency. *Ct* creatinine; *BP* blood pressure

and hence, the amount of sodium presented to the distal nephron where potassium excretion typically occurs, or to blockade of aldosterone production and release, or to a combination of both of these processes. ARBs may be an alternative in this setting since they cause smaller rises in potassium compared to ACE inhibitors [25].

References

1. Zisman LS, Abraham WT, Meixell GE, et al. Angiotensin II formation in the intact human heart. Predominance of the angiotensin-converting enzyme pathway. J Clin Invest. 1995;96(3):1490–8.
2. Garg R, Yusuf S. Overview of randomized trials of angiotensin-converting enzyme inhibitors on mortality and morbidity in patients with heart failure. Collaborative Group on ACE Inhibitor Trials. JAMA. 1995;273(18):1450–6.
3. Flather MD, Yusuf S, Kober L, et al. Long-term ACE-inhibitor therapy in patients with heart failure or left ventricular dysfunction: a systematic overview of data from individual patients. ACE-Inhibitor Myocardial Infarction Collaborative Group. Lancet. 2000;355(9215):1575–81.
4. Kober L, Torp-Pedersen C, Carlsen JE, et al. A clinical trial of the angiotensin-converting-enzyme inhibitor trandolapril in patients with left ventricular dysfunction after myocardial infarction. Trandolapril Cardiac Evaluation (TRACE) Study Group. N Engl J Med. 1995;333(25):1670–6.
5. Jong P, Demers C, McKelvie RS, et al. Angiotensin receptor blockers in heart failure: meta-analysis of randomized controlled trials. J Am Coll Cardiol. 2002;39(3):463–70.
6. Granger CB, McMurray JJ, Yusuf S, et al. Effects of candesartan in patients with chronic heart failure and reduced left-ventricular systolic function intolerant to angiotensin-converting-enzyme inhibitors: the CHARM-Alternative trial. Lancet. 2003;362(9386):772–6.

7. Lee VC, Rhew DC, Dylan M, et al. Meta-analysis: angiotensin-receptor blockers in chronic heart failure and high-risk acute myocardial infarction. Ann Intern Med. 2004;141(9): 693–704.

8. Pitt B, Segal R, Martinez FA, et al. Randomised trial of losartan versus captopril in patients over 65 with heart failure (Evaluation of Losartan in the Elderly Study, ELITE). Lancet. 1997;349(9054):747–52.

9. Pitt B, Poole-Wilson PA, Segal R, et al. Effect of losartan compared with captopril on mortality in patients with symptomatic heart failure: randomised trial—the Losartan Heart Failure Survival Study ELITE II. Lancet. 2000;355(9215):1582–7.

10. McKelvie RS, Yusuf S, Pericak D, et al. Comparison of candesartan, enalapril, and their combination in congestive heart failure: randomized evaluation of strategies for left ventricular dysfunction (RESOLVD) pilot study. The RESOLVD Pilot Study Investigators. Circulation. 1999;100(10):1056–64.

11. Cohn JN, Tognoni G. A randomized trial of the angiotensin-receptor blocker valsartan in chronic heart failure. N Engl J Med. 2001;345(23):1667–75.

12. McMurray JJ, Ostergren J, Swedberg K, et al. Effects of candesartan in patients with chronic heart failure and reduced left-ventricular systolic function taking angiotensin-converting-enzyme inhibitors: the CHARM-Added trial. Lancet. 2003;362(9386):767–71.

13. Pfeffer MA, Swedberg K, Granger CB, et al. Effects of candesartan on mortality and morbidity in patients with chronic heart failure: the CHARM-Overall programme. Lancet. 2003; 362(9386):759–66.

14. Yusuf S, Pfeffer MA, Swedberg K, et al. Effects of candesartan in patients with chronic heart failure and preserved left ventricular ejection fraction: the CHARM-Preserved Trial. Lancet. 2003;362(9386):777–81.

15. Kunz R, Friedrich C, Wolbers M, et al. Meta-analysis: effect of monotherapy and combination therapy with inhibitors of the renin angiotensin system on proteinuria in renal disease. Ann Intern Med. 2008;148(1):30–48.

16. Phillips CO, Kashani A, Ko DK, et al. Adverse effects of combination angiotensin II receptor blockers plus angiotensin-converting enzyme inhibitors for left ventricular dysfunction: a quantitative review of data from randomized clinical trials. Arch Intern Med. 2007;167(18): 1930–6.

17. Juurlink DN, Mamdani MM, Lee DS, et al. Rates of hyperkalemia after publication of the Randomized Aldactone Evaluation Study. N Engl J Med. 2004;351(6):543–51.

18. Pitt B, Bakris G, Ruilope LM, DiCarlo L, Mukherjee R. Serum potassium and clinical outcomes in the Eplerenone Post-Acute Myocardial Infarction Heart Failure Efficacy and Survival Study (EPHESUS). Circulation. 2008;118(16):1643–50.

19. Pitt B, Zannad F, Remme WJ, et al. The effect of spironolactone on morbidity and mortality in patients with severe heart failure. Randomized Aldactone Evaluation Study Investigators. N Engl J Med. 1999;341(10):709–17.

20. Pitt B. Effect of aldosterone blockade in patients with systolic left ventricular dysfunction: implications of the RALES and EPHESUS studies. Mol Cell Endocrinol. 2004;217(1–2): 53–8.

21. de Groote P, Isnard R, Assyag P, et al. Is the gap between guidelines and clinical practice in heart failure treatment being filled? Insights from the IMPACT RECO survey. Eur J Heart Fail. 2007;9(12):1205–11.

22. Hillege HL, Nitsch D, Pfeffer MA, et al. Renal function as a predictor of outcome in a broad spectrum of patients with heart failure. Circulation. 2006;113(5):671–8.

23. Bakris GL, Weir MR. Angiotensin-converting enzyme inhibitor-associated elevations in serum creatinine: is this a cause for concern? Arch Intern Med. 2000;160(5):685–93.

24. Knight EL, Glynn RJ, McIntyre KM, et al. Predictors of decreased renal function in patients with heart failure during angiotensin-converting enzyme inhibitor therapy: results from the studies of left ventricular dysfunction (SOLVD). Am Heart J. 1999;138(5 Pt 1):849–55.

25. Bakris GL, Siomos M, Richardson D, et al. ACE inhibition or angiotensin receptor blockade: impact on potassium in renal failure. VAL-K Study Group. Kidney Int. 2000;58(5):2084–92.

Hyperkalemia Risk and Treatment of Heart Failure

Julian Segura and Luis M. Ruilope

Introduction

Heart failure (HF) is a complex syndrome characterized by symptoms and signs related to inadequate perfusion of tissues during exercise and often to the retention of fluids, and represent the final common pathway for most primary cardiovascular diseases. Progressive ageing of the population, together with the significant reduction in mortality observed in the last years for the two main causes of HF, coronary artery disease and arterial hypertension, has been accompanied by a marked increase in its prevalence [1], so that HF is now considered a major public health problem [2]. Alterations in renal function play a key role in the pathophysiology of HF and are influenced by the treatment of this syndrome. Over the past few decades, the therapeutic approach for HF has undergone considerable change. The therapeutic management of HF can no longer be confined to the relief of symptoms, but is aimed to improve length and quality of life by preventing the progression of the disease [3]. In this concern, overwhelming evidence has demonstrated the efficacy of therapies antagonizing the neurohormonal activation, which is considered as a relevant component of HF treatment. However, the benefits of HF therapy do not come without some risk, and some increment in serum potassium (K^+), including the development of overt hyperkalemia (typically defined as a serum K^+ value in excess of 6.0 mEq/L), is to be expected [4].

This chapter briefly reviews the participation of the kidney in HF and the renal consequences of the treatment, with special emphasis on the risk of hyperkalemia and its management in daily clinical practice.

Originally published in Bakris, The Kidney in Heart Failure, ISBN: 978-1-4614-3693-5

J. Segura • L.M. Ruilope (✉)
Hypertension Unit, Nephrology Department, Hospital 12 de Octubre, Av. Córdoba s/n, 28041 Madrid, Spain
e-mail: ruilope@ad-hocbox.com

G.L. Bakris (ed.), *Managing the Kidney when the Heart is Failing*,
DOI 10.1007/978-1-4614-3691-1_3, © Springer Science+Business Media New York 2012

Renal Dysfunction and the Natural History of Heart Failure

Many years ago, it was proven that advanced degrees of HF are accompanied by marked reductions in renal plasma blood flow and glomerular filtration rate (GFR), which further contribute to implement sodium and water retention [5]. The development of progressive renal dysfunction is indeed a frequent complication in HF and represents the consequence of the combined effects of progressive decay in cardiac output and renal perfusion pressure, in conjunction with excess renal vasoconstriction. Advanced age, frequently present in patients with HF, contributes to facilitate the development of a decrease in GFR associated with the progression of HF. The progressive fall in GFR, which is observed in ages over 40 years in approximately two-thirds of subjects, particularly when hypertension is present [5] and the progressive renal vasoconstriction that accompanies ageing [6] are the main contributors to the worse renal adaptation to HF in elderly people. Recent data also indicate that patients suffering a myocardial infarction exhibit a more rapid decay in GFR with time when compared to "normals" [7, 8]. According to these data, factors predisposing the development of HF such as ageing, hypertension, and myocardial ischemia are also frequently accompanied by a diminished renal function, which in turn facilitates the development of renal function derangement if HF develops.

The degree and impact of renal dysfunction and its impact on outcomes in patients with HF are often underestimated. Most large outpatient chronic HF trials have excluded patients with renal dysfunction. Moreover, even when renal dysfunction is recognized, this diagnosis is often made solely on the basis of an elevated serum creatinine level. The National Kidney Foundation now advocates estimating GFR using the Modification of Diet in Renal Disease (MDRD) formula for all patients with renal insufficiency [9]. Because age, gender, race/ethnicity, and body habitus all significantly affect serum creatinine level, estimated GFR provides a more precise approximation of renal function than serum creatinine alone. In this sense, the ADHERE (Acute Decompensated HEart Failure National Registry) study is a large observational database of the clinical characteristics, management, and outcomes of patients hospitalized with acute decompensated HF, intended to determine the prevalence and severity of renal dysfunction at the time of hospital admission in patients with acute HF, and to relate the degree of renal dysfunction to treatments and inhospital outcomes [10]. As of August 2005, data from approximately 175,000 admissions at 280 participating hospitals had been entered into the registry. Overall, mean (±standard deviation) serum creatinine was 1.8 ± 1.6 mg/dL, mean BUN was 31.9 ± 21.0 mg/dL, and mean estimated GFR was $55.2 + 29.9$ mL/min/1.73 m^2. Interestingly, only 10,660 patients (9.0%) were classified as stage I (normal renal function); 32,423 patients (27.4%) were classified as stage II (mild renal dysfunction), 51,553 patients (43.5%) were classified as stage III (moderate renal dysfunction), 15,553 patients (13.1%) were classified as stage IV (severe renal dysfunction), and 8,276 patients (7.0%) were classified as stage V (kidney failure) [10]. This study concluded that renal dysfunction is frequent in patients admitted with acute HF, which is not adequately identified by serum creatinine level alone.

Interestingly, a decreased renal function is associated with a significant increment in mortality in HF [11, 12]. It has been suggested that a decreased GFR may represent a potent predictor of a lower survival in these patients [12]. The capacity of a deranged renal function to predict a poorer survival in HF patients recalls that described in essential hypertension and in the general population [13–16], where the finding of a small increase in serum creatinine or a decrease in GFR predicts a higher prevalence of cardiovascular events and death [17].

Moreover, the role of proteinuria in HF patients has not been extensively investigated. Proteinuria is a surrogate of structural kidney and vascular disease, and a marker for poor outcomes in diabetes mellitus, coronary artery disease, and hypertension, but the prognostic significance of proteinuria in HF has not been reported. In a secondary analysis of the Valsartan in HF Trial (Val-HeFT) database, the relationship between proteinuria and study end points controlling for other risk factors, including chronic kidney disease (CKD) has been examined [18]. A total of 5,010 patients were randomized in Val-HeFT, with 2,511 assigned to valsartan and 2,499 to placebo. There were 5,002 patients who had baseline estimated GFR values, and 4,958 patients had urinalysis at baseline. CKD, defined as estimated GFR <60 mL/min/1.73 m², was found in 2,916 patients (58%) at baseline. Dipstick proteinuria was positive in 405 patients (8.2%). There were 116 patients (2.3%) with proteinuria and no CKD, 2,601 (52%) with CKD and no proteinuria, and 289 (5.8%) with combined proteinuria and CKD. CKD was more prevalent in those with proteinuria [289/405 (72%) vs. 2,601/4,552 (48%), $P < 0.001$]. In this study, proteinuria was associated with an increased risk of mortality [unadjusted hazard ratio (HR) 1.76, 95% CI 1.46–2.13] and first morbid event (unadjusted HR 1.86, 95% CI 1.60–2.17). Figure 1 shows the unadjusted relationship between proteinuria and all-cause mortality and first morbid event in the subgroups with and without CKD. Patients with proteinuria had worse prognosis than those without proteinuria in both subgroups. Proteinuria was independently associated with mortality (HR 1.28, 95% CI 1.01–1.62, $P = 0.05$) and the first morbid event (HR 1.28, 95% CI 1.06–1.55, $P = 0.01$) after adjustment for other prognostic variables, including CKD. Patients with proteinuria had higher blood pressure and significantly lower serum albumin, which suggests perhaps a structural basis for proteinuria. These patients also had evidence of worse HF with more fluid retention. In particular, a much greater percentage had an elevated jugular venous pressure, peripheral edema, paroxysmal nocturnal dyspnea, third heart sound, and orthopnea, whereas mean plasma renin activity was much lower when proteinuria was present, which suggests a possible pathogenetic role of increased intravascular volume [18].

Pathophysiology of Hyperkalemia in Congestive Heart Failure

The pathophysiology of hyperkalemia in HF is typically multifactorial and related to variable contributions from two controlling processes: factors which preclude the normal inward cellular migration of K^+, and circumstances which interfere with the

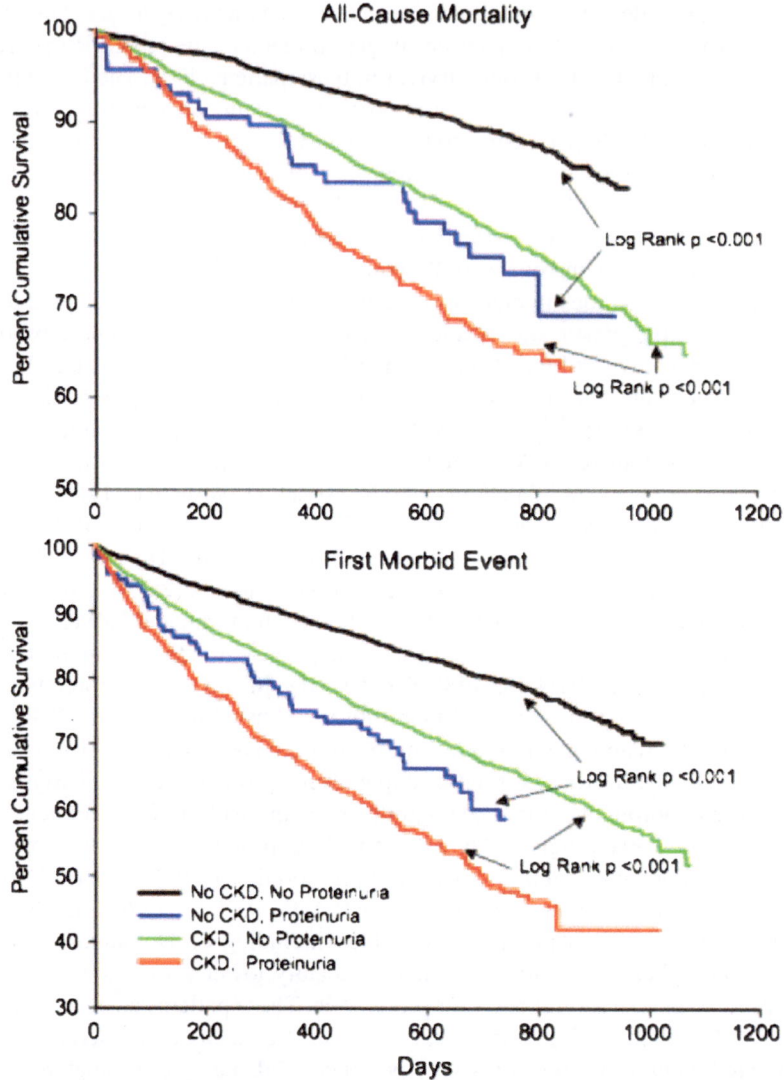

Fig. 1 Kaplan–Meier curves for time to death and first morbid event according to presence or absence of proteinuria and CKD. From [18]. Reprinted with kind permission from Lippincott Williams and Wilkins

external balance of K^+, as in the instance of a reduction in the renal clearance of K^+. Circumstances characterized by a reduction in the cellular entry of K^+ that are common in HF include: diabetes with concomitant insulin deficiency [19]; recurrent hyperosmolarity in association with hyperglycemia [20]; an increase in the dose of a β(beta) blocker [21]; and progressive metabolic acidosis [22]. Potassium excretion is diminished by two general mechanisms: firstly, a reduction in GFR, which is quite common and may be present despite a serum creatinine value within the "normal range" [23, 24]; and secondly, a reduction in K^+ excretion is often the result of pharmacotherapy, which includes angiotensin-converting enzyme (ACE) inhibitors, angiotensin receptor blockers (ARBs), and aldosterone receptor antagonists (ARAs), such as spironolactone or eplerenone [25]. Therein, K^+ excretion is reduced by a decrease in aldosterone production and/or interference on its renal effect.

ACE inhibitors and ARBs cause hyperkalemia by two mechanisms, including a fall in GFR and a reduction in aldosterone secretion. In HF patients, an ACE inhibitor-related decline in GFR can be abrupt, particularly when GFR is heavily dependent on angiotensin-II-mediated increases in efferent arteriolar tone [4]. A fall in GFR can occur at any time following initiation of ACE inhibitor therapy. Two patterns of GFR change exist:

- an immediate drop in GFR within days of therapy having begun, which generally reflects unrecognized volume contraction and/or micro- and macrovascular renal disease
- a drop in GFR in a HF patient with otherwise stable renal function that develops in conjunction with an intervening volume-contracting process, such as diarrhea or inadvertent over-diuresis.

The HF patient with significant systolic dysfunction can be quite sensitive to the blood pressure and/or GFR-reducing effects of ACE inhibition with changes occurring at very low doses. In such patients, choosing a nonaccumulating ACE inhibitor such as trandolapril or fosinopril, which present dual excretion through the liver and the kidney, may be preferable [4].

The sequence of events leading to a reduction in GFR with an ACE inhibitor can occur in a similar manner with ARB therapy. However, ARB therapy appears to be associated with a lesser magnitude effect on K^+ homeostasis. In a recent comparison (lisinopril vs. valsartan) in patients with renal insufficiency, treatment with lisinopril led to a greater increase in serum K^+ (0.28 mEq/L vs. 0.12 mEq/L). This difference was not explained by either differential change in renal function or plasma aldosterone concentration [26].

Hyperkalemia in Clinical Trials Including HF Patients

Trials Using ACE Inhibitors

Landmark clinical trials have demonstrated that ACE inhibitors reduce mortality and morbidity in patients with mild-to-severe HF [27–29]. The CONSENSUS (Cooperative North Scandinavian Enalapril Survival Study) trial evaluated the influence of an ACE inhibitor, enalapril (2.5–40 mg/day), on the prognosis of severe congestive HF in 253 patients randomly assigned to receive either placebo or

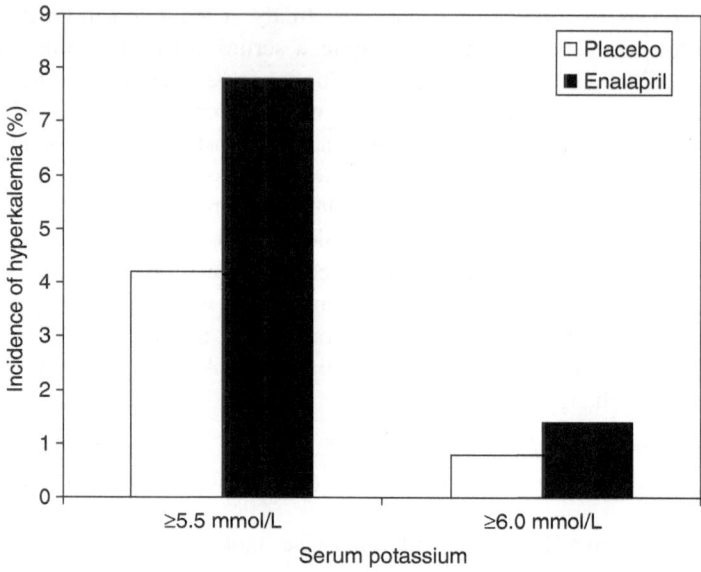

Fig. 2 Incidence of moderate (K$^+$ ≥5.5 mmol/L) and severe (K$^+$ ≥6.0 mmol/L) hyperkalemia in patients receiving enalapril or placebo in the SOLVD trials. Modified from [30]

enalapril [27]. The crude mortality at the end of 6 months was 26% in the enalapril group and 44% in the placebo group—a reduction of 40% ($P=0.002$). Mortality was reduced by 31% at 1 year ($P=0.001$). By the end of the study, there had been 68 deaths in the placebo group and 50 in the enalapril group—a reduction of 27% ($P=0.003$) [27]. The SOLVD (Studies of Left Ventricular Dysfunction) trials studied the effect of enalapril on total mortality and mortality from cardiovascular causes, the development of HF, and hospitalization for HF among 4,228 patients with ejection fractions of 0.35 or less who were not receiving drug treatment for HF [28, 29]. The total number of deaths and cases of HF was lower in the enalapril group than in the placebo group (630 vs. 818; risk reduction, 29%; 95% confidence interval, 21–36%; $P<0.001$). In addition, fewer patients given enalapril died or were hospitalized for HF (434 in the enalapril group vs. 518 in the placebo group; risk reduction, 20%; 95% confidence interval, 9–30%; $P<0.001$) [29].

Recently, a retrospective analysis of the SOLVD trial has been published to identify the factors associated with the development of hyperkalemia and to evaluate the impact of the definition of hyperkalemia on its incidence [30]. Baseline serum potassium was 4.3 ± 0.4 mmol/L. The mean follow-up was 2.7 ± 1.2 years. Serum potassium was measured a mean of 5.2 ± 2.9 times in each patients during this period. The incidence of hyperkalemia was 6.0% when using a definition of ≥5.5 mmol/L and 1.1% when using a cutoff value of ≥6.0 mmol/L. Hyperkalemia was statistically more frequent in the enalapril group compared with placebo, either when hyperkalemia was defined as potassium ≥5.5 mmol/L (7.8% vs 4.2%, $P<0.0001$) or as ≥6.0 mmol/L (1.4% vs 0.8%, $P<0.05$) (Fig. 2) [30]. The mean time to the first episode of hyperkalemia (≥5.5 mmol/L) was 1.0 ± 1.2 years (median 0.67 years). The peak incidence of hyperkalemia was greatest in the first 6 months [30]. Most cases of hyperkalemia occurred once patients had been titrated to the target dose of enalapril (20 mg/day, 66.5%), whereas a more limited number occurred at lower daily doses (2.5 mg/day 4.9%, 5 mg/day 11.0%, 10 mg/day 17.5%) [30]. In the multivariate analysis, using serum creatinine levels to estimate renal function, predictors of hyperkalemia included randomization to enalapril, baseline serum creatinine, baseline serum potassium, a history of atrial fibrillation, a history of diabetes, NYHA functional class III/IV, and the use of loop diuretics [30]. Focusing on renal function, the risk of hyperkalemia was significantly increased only in patients with moderate (creatinine clearance 30–59 mL/min, $P < 0.0001$) and severe dysfunction (creatinine clearance <30 mL/min, $P = 0.0002$), compared with patients with a normal function (creatinine clearance >90 mL/min). Mild renal dysfunction had no impact on the risk of hyperkalemia (creatinine clearance 60–89 mL/min, $P = 0.48$), suggesting a threshold effect for the risk of hyperkalemia development [30].

Trials Using ARBs

The effects of ARBs have also been evaluated in patients with HF. The Optimal Trial in Myocardial Infarction with the Angiotensin II Antagonist Losartan 56 (OPTIMAAL) involved 5,477 patients with acute MI and evidence of HF or left ventricular dysfunction. Patients were randomized to receive losartan or captopril. After 2.7 years of follow-up, the reduction in risk for all-cause mortality did not differ significantly between losartan and captopril. Losartan was associated with a significantly lower risk for CV death than captopril, although only low-dose losartan was used [31]. A significant between-group difference was detected for serum potassium, increasing from 4.16 to 4.36 mmol/L in patients treated with losartan, and from 4.16 to 4.38 mmol/L in those receiving captopril ($P < 0.01$) [31]. The Valsartan Heart Failure Trial 58 (Val-HeFT) found no significant reduction in mortality rate with ARB therapy in 5,010 ACE inhibitor-treated patients with HF. Compared with placebo, valsartan was associated with a significant reduction in the risk for the combined end point of CV morbidity and mortality, defined as hospital admission for HF, cardiac arrest, and need for intravenous inotropic or vasodilator therapy, largely as a result of the reduced risk for HF hospitalization [32]. The mean change in the serum potassium concentration was an increase of 0.12 mmol/L with valsartan and a decrease of 0.07 mmol/L with placebo ($P < 0.001$) [32].

The CHARM (Candesartan in Heart Failure-Assessment of Reduction in Mortality and Morbidity) Program investigated the impact of treatment with the ARB candesartan, both alone and in combination with an ACE inhibitor, across a broad spectrum of symptomatic HF patients, including those with both depressed and preserved left ventricular ejection fraction (LVEF) and those treated with various combinations of neurohumoral antagonists [33]. Patients were enrolled into one of the three trials according to LVEF higher than 40% (CHARM-Preserved, $n = 3.023$), 40% or lower and treated with an ACE inhibitor (CHARM-Added, $n=2.548$), or 40% or lower and not treated with an ACE inhibitor due to prior intolerance (CHARM-Alternative, $n=2.028$) [34–36]. CHARM-Alternative evaluated effectiveness in 2,028 patients who were unable to tolerate ACE inhibitor therapy over a mean follow-up period of 33.7 months. In this population, candesartan significantly reduced the incidence of CV-related death or hospital admission for HF compared with placebo [36]. An analysis of the incidence and predictors of hyperkalemia in the CHARM Program has been recently published [37]. The incidence of clinically important hyperkalemia according to treatment assigned in the composite CHARM Program and each of the component trials is summarized in Table 1. Hyperkalemia was most common for both placebo- and candesartan-treated patients in CHARM-Added (2.9% placebo, 8.4% candesartan) in which patients were treated concurrently with an ACE inhibitor. In CHARM-Alternative, these percentages were 1.5% and 4.0%, respectively [37].

Independent of treatment assignment in the CHARM-Overall study, the risk of hyperkalemia increased with male gender, age ≥75 years, diabetes, background use of ACE inhibitors or spironolactone, baseline creatinine ≥2.0 mg/dL, and baseline potassium ≥5.0 mmol/L. The greatest relative risk increase for hyperkalemia was seen in patients with baseline renal insufficiency, whether or not they received candesartan (OR=4.1, 95% CI 2.4–7.3 for creatinine ≥2.0 mg/dL vs. <2.0 mg/dL). Serious hyperkalemia events (associated with hospitalization or death) were also more common in this group (OR=3.5, 95% CI 1.5–7.9 for creatinine ≥2.0 mg/dL vs. <2.0 mg/dL). Notably, the incidence of hyperkalemia in patients with creatinine ≥2 mg/dL receiving placebo (10%) was more than twice that of patients with creatinine <2 mg/dL receiving candesartan (4.9%) [37].

In multivariable Cox models containing treatment assignment, age ≥75 years, gender, blood pressure, diabetes, ACE inhibitor use, spironolactone use, nonsteroidal antiinflammatory drug use, ejection fraction <40%, beta-blocker use, and loop diuretic use, assignment to candesartan, male gender, age ≥75 years, diabetes, and background use of ACE inhibitors or spironolactone remained clinically important predictors of hyperkalemia (Table 2). When the model was extended to include baseline creatinine and potassium for the subset of 2,675 patients in whom laboratory data were available, the effects of gender and diabetes were attenuated, but renal function, baseline potassium, age ≥75 years, baseline use of ACE inhibitors or spironolactone, and assignment to candesartan were still relevant predictors [37].

It is often anticipated that with increasing age and associated comorbidities, tolerability to therapy with inhibitors of the renin–angiotensin system is lessened because of the decreased renal function, hyperkalemia, and hypotension. These arguments are also often used to not titrate HF drugs to the high doses recommended by guidelines. A recent analysis from the CHARM study examined the effect of age on clinical outcomes, including mortality, hospitalization, and adverse drug effects, and to determine whether the therapeutic response to candesartan was influenced by increasing age [38]. This study showed that, in chronic HF, increasing age was associated with different patient characteristics at baseline, and a worse prognosis. However, the relative benefit from candesartan in older patients was

Table 1 Incidence of clinically important hyperkalemia in CHARM

	Placebo		Candesartan		
	n/N (%)	Per 1,000 patient-years	n/N (%)	Per 1,000 patient-years	OR (95% CI)
CHARM-Alternative	15/1.015 (1.5%)	5.9	40/1.013 (4.0%)	15.4	2.7 (1.5–5.0)
CHARM-Added	37/1.272 (2.9%)	10.1	107/1.276 (8.4%)	29.1	3.1 (2.1–4.5)
CHARM-Preserved	18/1.509 (1.2%)	4.1	50/1.514 (3.3%)	11.5	2.8 (1.6–4.9)
CHARM-Overall	70/3.796 (1.8%)	6.6	197/3.803 (5.2%)	18.5	2.9 (2.2–3.9)

Modified from [37]

Table 2 Multivariable HRs
for clinically important
hyperkalemia in CHARM

Parameter	HR (95% CI)
Multivariable model excluding potassium and creatinine (full CHARM cohort, $n = 7.599$)	
Treatment assignment	**2.8 (2.2–3.7)**
Age ≥75 years	**1.7 (1.3–2.3)**
Diabetes	**2.0 (1.6–2.6)**
ACE inhibitor use	**1.8 (1.1–3.1)**
Spironolactone use	**1.8 (1.3–2.3)**
Male gender	**1.4 (1.0–2.0)**
Multivariable model including potassium and creatinine (North American cohort, $n = 2.675$)	
Treatment assignment	**2.1 (1.4–3.1)**
Age ≥75 years	**1.5 (1.0–2.3)**
Diabetes	1.2 (0.8–1.7)
ACE inhibitor use	**2.2 (1.0–4.6)**
Spironolactone use	1.6 (1.0–2.4)
Male gender	1.3 (0.8–1.9)
Creatinine ≥2.0	**3.4 (2.1–5.7)**
Potassium ≥5.0	**2.6 (1.7–4.0)**

Variables in bold were significant at the $P < 0.05$ level
From [37]. Reprinted with kind permission from Elsevier

similar to that observed in younger patients. Tolerability of candesartan, relative to placebo, was similar across all age ranges at the doses achieved. The proportion of patients discontinuing candesartan compared with placebo for these three adverse effects was similar across all age groups, with no interaction between age and treatment, except for the risk of increased serum creatinine, which was relatively lower in the most elderly [38].

Interestingly, patients with CKD obtain greater absolute benefit in long-term outcomes than do those without CKD [18]. The number needed to treat with valsartan to prevent one morbid event was substantially less for patients with underlying CKD than for those with normal underlying kidney function. These findings highlight the clinical importance of several studies that have shown an underutilization of ACEIs and ARBs in HF patients with underlying CKD.

High ARB doses could achieve improved clinical benefits, through more complete inhibition of angiotensin effects at the AT1 receptor or increased stimulation of the AT2 receptor [39]. Recently, the Heart failure Endpoint evaluation of Angiotensin II Antagonist Losartan (HEAAL) study compared clinical outcomes in patients with HF, reduced LVEF, and intolerance to ACE inhibitors who were randomly assigned to a high (150 mg) or low (50 mg) daily dose of losartan [40]. This study hypothesized that incremental losartan dosing would reduce the risk of the primary combined endpoint of death or admission for HF. Overall, 1,927 patients were randomly assigned to losartan 150 mg daily and 1,919 to losartan 50 mg daily. The reported reasons for ACE inhibitor intolerance were cough ($n = 3,294$, 86%), symptomatic hypotension (269, 7%), gastrointestinal upset (193, 5%), rash (97, 3%), taste disturbance (86, 2%), hyperkalemia (56, 1%), and azotemia (39, 1%), with some patients having more than one of these symptoms. Losartan 150 mg daily significantly reduced the rate of the primary endpoint compared with losartan 50 mg. About 828 (43%) patients in the 150 mg group and 889 (46%) in the 50 mg group died or were admitted for HF (HR 0.90, 95% CI 0.82–0.99; $P=0.027$). At 12 months, serum potassium increased by a mean of 0.02 mmol/L in the 150 mg group and decreased by 0.01 mmol/L in the 50 mg group ($P=0.03$ between groups). Serum potassium concentrations were 6·0 mmol/L or greater in 20 (1%) patients in the 150 mg group and in 14 (1%) in the 50 mg group ($P=0.32$). Estimated GFR was 6.1 mL/min/1.73 m² lower at 12 months than at baseline for the 150 mg group and 1.9 mL/min/1.73 m² lower for the 50 mg group ($P<0.0001$ between groups). At 12 months, serum creatinine at least doubled from baseline in 19 (1%) patients in the 150 mg group and nine (<1%) in the 50 mg group ($P=0.06$). At the end of the study, 195 (2.79 per 100 person-years) and 131 (1.87 per 100 person-years) developed hyperkalemia in the 150 and 50 mg groups, respectively ($P=0.0004$), but discontinuation of masked medication was infrequent (9 patients, 0.12 per 100 person-years, and 4 patients, 0.05 per 100 person-years, respectively) ($P=0.20$) [40]. In agreement with previous studies, these authors conclude that blood pressure, serum electrolytes, and renal function should be monitored carefully during ARB up-titration, and the clinical implications of changes in any of these variables should be weighed against the potential outcome benefits that are achievable with an increased ARB dose [40].

Trials Using ACE Inhibitors Plus ARBs

Dual suppression of the renin–angiotensin–aldosterone system with combination therapy that includes ACE inhibitors and ARBs is gaining interest among HF experts [41].

In CHARM-Added, candesartan was added to the regimen of 2,548 patients with HF and LVEF ≤40% who were already receiving ACE inhibitors. Candesartan was significantly more effective than placebo in reducing the RR for the primary combined end point of CV-related death and hospital admission for congestive HF, as well as for each component of the composite end point [34]. In the Valsartan in Acute Myocardial Infarction Trial (VALIANT), 14,703 patients with acute myocardial infarction and clinical or radiologic signs of HF, LVD, or both were randomized to receive valsartan 20 mg, captopril 6.25 mg, or valsartan plus captopril. All-cause mortality was not improved, the occurrence of CV end points was not reduced, and adverse events increased with the combination of valsartan and captopril compared with captopril alone [42]. Despite the initial enthusiasm for combination ARBs plus ACE inhibitors as a viable therapeutic option for subsets of patients with symptomatic left ventricular dysfunction, current guidelines recommending pharmacotherapy in patients with HF have not endorsed this approach [43]. Moreover, concerns about adverse effects including severe or life-threatening hyperkalemia persist [26, 44]

Table 3 Results for worsening renal function and hyperkalemia with combination ACE inhibitors plus ARBs

	Worsening renal function, n/N (%)		Hyperkalemia, n/N (%)	
	Intervention	Control	Intervention	Control
VALIANT	232/4,885 (4.8)	148/4,909 (3.0)	57/4,885 (1.2)	43/4,909 (0.9)
CHARM-Added	100/1,276 (7.8)	52/1,272 (4.1)	44/1,276 (3.5)	9/1,272 (0.7)
Val-HEFT	27/2,326 (1.1)	4/2,318 (0.4)	–	–
RESOLVD	2/332 (0.6)	0/109 (0.0)	–	–
Subtotals				
Chronic HF	128/3,934 (3.3)	55/3,699 (1.5)	44/1,276 (3.5)	9/1,272 (0.7)
RR (95% CI)	2.17 (1.59–2.97)		4.87 (2.39–9.94)	
AMI with LVD	232/4,885 (4.8)	148/4,909 (3.0)	57/4,885 (1.2)	43/4,909 (0.9)
RR (95% CI)	1.61 (1.31–1.98)		1.33 (0.90–1.98)	
Pooled cohort	360/8,819 (4.1)	203/8,608 (2.4)	101/6,161 (1.6)	52/6,181 (0.8)
RR (95% CI)	1.76 (1.49–2.09)		2.46 (0.68–8.87)	

Modified from [41]

and may limit the application of this strategy [40]. In fact, it has been recently published an analysis to characterize and quantify the risk of adverse effects of combination ACE inhibitor plus ARB therapy in patients with chronic HF or acute myocardial infarction with symptomatic left ventricular dysfunction, particularly the associated risk of worsening renal function or development of hyperkalemia [41]. Table 3 shows a summary of the results for worsening renal function and hyperkalemia in trials combining ACE inhibitors plus ARBs. Worsening renal function (defined as an increase in serum creatinine level >0.5 mg/dL, up to a doubling over baseline values) was significantly increased with combination ARB plus ACE inhibitor therapy vs. control treatment in patients with chronic HF, and there was a significant increase in the risk of hyperkalemia with serum potassium level of 5.5 mEq/L or greater. Combination of ARB plus ACE inhibitor therapy vs. control treatment was also associated with a significant increase in the risk of worsening renal function in AMI with symptomatic left ventricular dysfunction and a nonsignificant increase in the risk of hyperkalemia [41].

Trials Using ARAs

Spironolactone and eplerenone have emerged as significant adjunctive treatments for HF. The Randomized Aldactone Evaluation Study (RALES) demonstrated that treatment with spironolactone substantially reduced morbidity and mortality in patients with severe HF [45]. Hyperkalemia developed in only a few patients (2%) in the active-treatment group in RALES. The low incidence of hyperkalemia may reflect unusually close laboratory monitoring, restriction of other drugs that cause hyperkalemia, or exclusion of patients with advanced renal disease or mild hyperkalemia at baseline. In fact, a population-based time-series analysis published in 2004 demonstrated an increase in spironolactone use and hyperkalemia-associated morbidity and mortality at the population level [46].

There are several reasons explaining why hyperkalemia is a more common occurrence in clinical practice than it was in the carefully controlled setting of RALES: physicians may not monitor potassium levels closely in patients receiving spironolactone, may neglect baseline attributes that predispose patients to hyperkalemia (e.g., diabetes mellitus), and may overlook conditions that develop during therapy (e.g., renal dysfunction). Moreover, they may prescribe inappropriately high doses of spironolactone or other medications that contribute to hyperkalemia. Some patients may purposefully increase their dietary potassium intake, as is often recommended during treatment with diuretics such as furosemide. Finally, physicians may extend the RALES findings to patients who, unlike the patients in that study, do not have left ventricular systolic dysfunction (e.g., those with diastolic dysfunction or cor pulmonale) [46].

In the Eplerenone Post-acute myocardial infarction Heart Failure Efficacy and Survival Study (EPHESUS), other ARA, eplerenone, significantly reduced the morbidity and mortality associated with left ventricular dysfunction and congestive HF in the postmyocardial infarction patient when compared with placebo [47]. At 1 year into this study, potassium levels increased in both the placebo (0.2 mEq/L) and active therapy groups (0.3 mEq/L), $P < 0.001$. Serious hyperkalemia (serum potassium concentration ≥ 6.0 mEq/L) was more common in eplerenone-treated patients (5.5%) compared with placebo (3.9%). In EPHESUS, the incidence of hyperkalemia was increased in patients with a creatinine clearance below 50 mL/min [eplerenone (10.1%); placebo (5.9%)]. In patients with a baseline creatinine clearance >50 mL/min, the corresponding rates were 4.6% and 3.5%, respectively. Of note, eplerenone reduced the risk of hypokalemia, which was twice as high as the risk of serious hyperkalemia [47].

Trials Using Direct Renin Inhibitors

Direct renin inhibitors (DRIs) offer another pharmacologically distinct way to suppress the renin–angiotensin–aldosterone system (RAAS), with the theoretical advantages of blocking an enzyme with only one known substrate (angiotensinogen), inhibiting the rate-limiting step in the renin–angiotensin–aldosterone cascade, and reducing synthesis of all subsequent components of the cascade [48]. As with ARBs, DRIs may offer an alternative to an ACE inhibitor or could be used in combination with an ACE inhibitor (or ARB). The rationale for the latter approach is that ACE inhibitors (and ARBs) induce a compensatory rise in renin and downstream RAAS components that may eventually overcome their RAAS-blocking effect. A DRI should block this compensatory increase in RAAS activity. Conversely, the addition of an ACE inhibitor (or ARB) to a DRI may be valuable in view of the possibility of nonrenin production of angiotensin I through enzymes such as cathepsin D and tonin [49]. Until recently, the introduction of renin inhibitors into clinical practice was limited by the low oral bioavailability, poor efficacy, short duration of action, and high cost of chemical synthesis of previous compounds. These problems have been overcome with the development of the new, orally active, nonpeptide, specific renin

Table 4 Biochemical abnormalities in the ALOFT study

Biochemical abnormalities, n (%)	Placebo ($n = 146$)	Aliskiren ($n = 156$)
Creatinine (μmol/L)		
>177	8 (5.6)	11 (7.1)
>265	3 (2.1)	0 (0.0)
Potassium (mmol/L)		
>5.5	12 (8.3)	13 (8.3)
≥6.0	6 (4.2)	3 (1.9)

Modified from [51]

inhibitor, aliskiren. Seed et al. show the neurohumoral effects of administration of aliskiren to patient with chronic HF in comparison with placebo and with an effective dose of ramipril [50]. They studied 27 patients (3 female) and all had been taking an ACE inhibitor prior to randomization. Aliskiren was at least as effective at suppressing the RAAS as the ACE inhibitor ramipril over a 6-week period. This effect was apparent acutely, where 1 week of treatment with 75 mg of aliskiren reduced plasma angiotensin II concentrations, in contrast to 5 mg of ramipril. This effect was also apparent over the subsequent 5 weeks of treatment, where 75–300 mg of aliskiren more clearly reduced angiotensin II than ramipril 5–10 mg [50]. Taking into account the clinical success of the established pharmacological approaches for RAAS inhibition in cardiovascular and noncardiovascular diseases, it must be of interest to examine the clinical effects of renin inhibition, especially in chronic HF.

Recently, it has been published the Aliskiren Observation of Heart Failure Treatment (ALOFT) study, intended to analyze the effects of adding the DRI aliskiren to an ACE inhibitor in patients with HF [51]. Three hundred and two patients were included, all had a history of hypertension according to the inclusion criteria, but baseline seated blood pressure was 129 ± 17.4 mmHg systolic and 77 ± 9.5 mmHg diastolic. Although a low LVEF was not an inclusion criterion, 79% of patients had an LVEF ≤40%, and the mean ± SD LVEFs was $31 \pm 5.5\%$. Thirty-five percent of patients had a history of diabetes mellitus. Most patients were in New York Heart Association functional class II (61%) or III (38%) and were treated with neurohumoral blockers. Ninety-four percent were treated with an ACE inhibitor (or ARB) and beta-blocker and 32% with an aldosterone antagonist as well. Of the 302 patients randomized, 277 (92%) completed the double-blind treatment phase. Eleven (7.5%) placebo-treated and 14 (9.0%) aliskiren-treated patients discontinued the use of the study drug prematurely. Of these, two placebo-treated and one aliskiren-treated patient died, and four placebo-treated and seven aliskiren-treated patients discontinued the use of the drug because of an adverse event. Discontinuations related to the primary end point (renal dysfunction, symptomatic hypotension, or hyperkalemia) and worsening HF occurred in four aliskiren-treated patients (two hypotension, one hyperkalemia, and one worsening HF) and three placebo-treated patients (all due to worsening HF). There were no statistically significant differences in renal function assessment (Table 4). In conclusion, this study shows that the addition of aliskiren 150 mg/d to standard therapy for HF that includes an ACE inhibitor (or ARB), a beta-blocker, and an aldosterone antagonist, if indicated, appeared to be well tolerated, with only slightly (but not statistically significantly) higher rates of hypotension and hyperkalemia.

Approach to Hyperkalemia in HF Patients

ACE inhibitors, ARBs, and ARAs all have well-established capacities to diminish mortality in HF. Therefore, even in patients liable to develop hyperkalemia, every effort should be made to implement and/or continue the use of these compounds [4]. There are several recommendations to avoid or reduce hyperkalemia.

Dietary Interventions

Dietary changes including restriction of potassium intake should be preemptively instituted, specially using a combination of two blockers of RAAS. This maneuver alone is often sufficient to forestall the onset of hyperkalemia. In this regard, the patient should be questioned relative to the use of salt substitutes. By default, HF patients may view a salt substitute as an acceptable seasoning agent, being that they are otherwise routinely restricted in their intake of sodium [4]. Potassium supplements should be cautiously administered. In the management of moderate hyperkalemia, administration of binding resins to reduce potassium intestinal absorption should be a valuable tool [52].

Laboratory Monitoring for Serum Potassium and Renal Function

A recent study has demonstrated that only two-thirds of the patients had serum laboratory values obtained in the first 3 months after initiating spironolactone. The remaining 34% were prescribed spironolactone by a physician without any follow-up monitoring [53]. This fact contrasts with laboratory procedures in RALES, where patients initially treated with spironolactone had serum potassium and creatinine concentrations measured at 4, 8, and 12 weeks, and then every 3 months for up to 1 year. Periodic surveillance of serum potassium and creatinine (e.g., at baseline, within 1–2 weeks of a change in drug dosing, and at least annually thereafter) is critically important to limiting adverse events [37, 44].

Recommendations Involving RAAS Inhibitors

The onset of hyperkalemia may call for short-term discontinuation of either ACE inhibitor or ARB therapy until the issue of hyperkalemia can be resolved; thereafter, low-dose ACE inhibitor or ARB therapy can be cautiously reintroduced. Titration to the desired end dose of either drug class should only occur in tandem with periodic assessment of serum potassium values [4]. The duration of drug effect may be a pertinent consideration in the development of hyperkalemia in the HF patient, in that short-acting (or low-dose) ACE inhibitor therapy is less apt to produce hyperkalemia [4].

When combination therapy with ACE inhibitors or ARBs and an ARA is employed, patients should always be advised as to the risk inherent to the potential development of volume-depletion and its consequences. Frequently, volume contraction and the accompanying reduction in renal function provoke a dramatic and often life-threatening change in serum potassium [54]. When difficult-to-treat hyperkalemia occurs in the HF patient receiving an ARA, the dose of each compound can be empirically reduced or the same dose can be given on an every-other-day basis. However, there is little information available that addresses the survival benefits of spironolactone or eplerenone at doses less than 25 and 50 mg/day, respectively. If spironolactone therapy is the basis for hyperkalemia development, then an empiric switch to eplerenone can be considered based on eplerenone half-life being shorter. However, head-to-head studies in HF comparing equivalent doses of eplerenone and spironolactone for hyperkalemia risk have yet to be undertaken. Finally, combining spironolactone or eplerenone with a loop (potassium-losing) diuretic alone, or together with metolazone, may preempt the development of hyperkalemia [4].

Diuretic Use

Loop and thiazide-type diuretics should be carefully used in the setting of HF and hyperkalemia, whereas an increase in urine flow rate may facilitate urinary potassium excretion, an excessive diuretic response with accompanying volume-depletion or contraction can reduce urinary potassium excretion. If diuretic-related volume losses are extreme enough, GFR may fall and urinary sodium excretion drop. The latter can importantly reduce urinary potassium excretion [4].

Conclusions

Potassium surveillance in HF mandates a careful estimate of the level of renal function and a baseline serum potassium determination before therapy is added, and especially for combined therapy. Periodic surveillance of serum potassium and creatinine is critically important to limiting adverse events.

The subset of older HF patients who have moderate or severe renal dysfunction, those with high serum potassium at baseline, and those who receive combination RAAS antagonists are particularly vulnerable, necessitating even closer monitoring.

Strategies to limit the toxicity of RAAS antagonists, such as restriction of potassium intake, elimination of drugs that may impair renal potassium excretion, and careful assessment of baseline renal function to identify those at especially high risk (e.g., eGFR < 45 mL/min/1.73 m^2), should be routinely considered.

The risk of hyperkalemia in HF patients receiving RAAS blockers should always be viewed in the context of survival benefits. Taken into account previous recommendations, hyperkalemia risk can be kept to a minimum and the attendant benefits of the therapy realized.

References

1. US Department of Health and Human Services. Heart failure: evaluation and care of patients with left ventricular systolic dysfunction. Clinical Practice Guidelines no. 11, AHCPR publication no. 94-0612, June 1994.
2. Kannel WB, Ho K, Thom T. Changing epidemiological features of cardiac failure. Br Heart J. 1994;72 Suppl 2:S3–9.
3. Cohn JN. The management of chronic heart failure. N Engl J Med. 1996;335:490–8.
4. Sica DA, Hess M. Pharmacotherapy in congestive heart therapy: aldosterone receptor antagonism: interface with hyperkalemia in heart failure. Congest Heart Fail. 2004;10:259–64.
5. Lindeman RD, Tobin JD, Shock NW. Association between blood pressure and the rate of decline in renal function with age. Kidney Int. 1984;26:861–8.
6. Ruilope LM, Lahera V, Rodicio JL, Romero JC. Are renal hemodynamics a key factor in the development and maintenance of essential hypertension? Hypertension. 1994;23:3–9.
7. Eijkelkamp WB, de Graeff PA, van Veldhuisen DJ, et al. Prevention of Renal and Vascular End-Stage Disease (PREVEND) Study Group. Effect of first myocardial ischemic event on renal function. Am J Cardiol. 2007;100:7–12.
8. Muntner P, Coresh J, Powe NR, Klag MJ. The contribution of increased diabetes prevalence and improved myocardial infarction and stroke survival to the increase in treated end-stage renal disease. J Am Soc Nephrol. 2003;14:1568–77.
9. Levey AS, Coresh J, Balk E, et al. National Kidney Foundation practice guidelines for chronic kidney disease: evaluation, classification, and stratification. Ann Intern Med. 2003;139:137–47.
10. Heywood JT, Fonarow GC, Costanzo MR, Mathur VS, Wigneswaran JR, Wynne J, for the ADHERE scientific advisory committee and investigators. High prevalence of renal dysfuncion and its impact on outcome in 118,465 patients hospitalized with acute decompensated heart failure: a report from the ADHERE database. J Cardiac Fail. 2007;13:422–30.
11. Ljungman S, Kjekshus J, Swedberg K, for the Consensus Trial Group. Renal function in severe congestive heart failure during treatment with enalapril. Am J Cardiol. 1992;70:479–87.
12. Hillege HL, Girbes AR, de Kam PJ, et al. Renal function, neurohumoral activation and survival in patients with chronic heart failure. Circulation. 2000;102:203–10.
13. Shulman NB, Ford CE, Hall WD, et al. Prognostic value of serum creatinine and effect of treatment of hypertension on renal function. Results from the hypertension detection and follow-up program. Hypertension. 1989;13(Suppl I):I80–93.
14. Ruilope LM, Campo C, Rodriguez-Artalejo F, Lahera V, Garcia-Robles R, Rodicio JL. Blood pressure and renal function: therapeutic implications. J Hypertens. 1996;14:1259–63.
15. Ruilope LM, Salvetti A, Jamerson K, et al. Renal function and intensive lowering of blood pressure in hypertensive participants of the hypertension optimal treatment (HOT) study. J Am Soc Nephrol. 2001;12:218–25.
16. Culleton BF, Larson MG, Wilson PWF, Evans JC, Parfrey PS, Levy D. Cardiovascular disease and mortality in a community-based cohort with mild renal insufficiency. Kidney Int. 1999;56:2214–9.

17. Ruilope LM, Barrios V, Volpe M. Renal implications of the renin-angiotensin-aldosterone system blockade in heart failure. J Hypertens. 2000;18:1545–51.

18. Anand IS, Bishu K, Rector TS, Ishani A, Kuskowski MA, Cohn JN. Proteinuria, chronic kidney disease and the effect of an angiotensin receptor blocker in addition to an angiotensin-converting enzyme inhibitor in patients with moderate to severe heart failure. Circulation. 2009;120:1577–84.

19. DeFronzo RA, Sherwin RS, Felig P, et al. Nonuremic diabetic hyperkalemia: possible role of insulin deficiency. Arch Intern Med. 1977;137:842–3.

20. Bratusch-Marrain PR, DeFronzo RA. Impairment of insulin-mediated glucose metabolism by hyperosmolarity in man. Diabetes. 1983;32:1028–34.

21. Rosa RM, Silva P, Young JB, et al. Adrenergic modulation of extrarenal potassium disposal. N Engl J Med. 1980;302:431–4.

22. Kurtzman NA, Gonzalez J, DeFronzo R, et al. A patient with hyperkalemia and metabolic acidosis. Am J Kidney Dis. 1990;15:333–56.

23. Cody RJ, Ljungman S, Covit AB, et al. Regulation of glomerular filtration rate in chronic congestive heart failure patients. Kidney Int. 1988;34:361–7.

24. Obialo CI, Ofili EO, Mirza T. Hyperkalemia in congestive heart failure patients aged 63 to 85 years with subclinical renal disease. Am J Cardiol. 2002;90:663–5.

25. Lawson DH, O'Connor PC, Jick H. Drug attributed alterations in potassium handling in congestive cardiac failure. Eur J Clin Pharmacol. 1982;23:21–5.

26. Bakris GL, Siomos M, Richardson D, et al. ACE inhibition or angiotensin receptor blockade: impact on potassium in renal failure. Kidney Int. 2000;58:2084–92.

27. The CONSENSUS Trial Study Group. Effects of enalapril on mortality in severe congestive heart failure. Results of the Cooperative North Scandinavian Enalapril Survival Study (CONSENSUS). N Engl J Med. 1987;316:1429–35.

28. The SOLVD Investigators. Effect of enalapril on survival in patients with reduced left ventricular ejection fractions and congestive heart failure. N Engl J Med. 1991;325:293–302.

29. The SOLVD Investigators. Effect of enalapril on mortality and the development of heart failure in asymptomatic patients with reduced left ventricular ejection fractions. N Engl J Med. 1992;327:685–91.

30. de Denus S, Tardif JC, White M, et al. Quantification of the risk and predictors of hyperkalemia in patients with left ventricular dysfunction: a retrospective analysis of the Studies of Left Ventricular Dysfunction (SOLVD) trials. Am Heart J. 2006;152:705–12.

31. Dickstein K, Kjekshus J, for the OPTIMAAL Steering Committee of the OPTIMAAL Study Group. Effects of losartan and captopril on mortality and morbidity in high-risk patients after acute myocardial infarction: The OPTIMAAL randomised trial. Optimal Trial in Myocardial Infarction with Angiotensin II Antagonist Losartan. Lancet. 2002;360:752–60.

32. Cohn JN, Tognoni G, for the Valsartan Heart Failure Trial Investigators. A randomized trial of the angiotensin-receptor blocker valsartan in chronic heart failure. N Engl J Med. 2001;345:1667–75.

33. Pfeffer MA, Sweberg K, Granger CB, et al. CHARM Investigators and Committees. Effects of candesartan on mortality and morbidity in patients with chronic heart failure: the CHARM-Overall programme. Lancet 2003;362:759–66.

34. McMurray JJ, Ostergren J, Swedberg K, et al. CHARM Investigators and Committees. Effects of candesartan in patients with chronic heart failure and reduced left ventricular systolic function treated with an ACE inhibitor: the CHARM-Added trial. Lancet. 2003;362:767–71.

35. Granger CB, McMurray JJ, Yusuf S, et al. CHARM Investigators and Committees. Effects of candesartan in patients with chronic heart failure and reduced left ventricular systolic function and intolerant to ACE inhibitors: the CHARM-Alternative trial. Lancet. 2003;362:772–6.

36. Yusuf S, Pfeffer MA, Swedberg K, et al. CHARM Investigators and Committees. Effects of candesartan in patients with chronic heart failure and preserved left ventricular systolic function: the CHARM-Preserved trial. Lancet. 2003;362:777–81.

37. Desai AS, Swedberg K, McMurray JJV, et al. Incidence and predictors of hyperkalemia in patients with heart failure. J Am Coll Cardiol. 2007;50:1959–66.

38. Cohen-Solal A, McMurray JJV, Swedberg K, et al. Benefits and safety of candesartan treatment in heart failure are independent of age: insights from the Candesartan in Heart failure-Assessment of Reduction in Mortality and morbidity programme. Eur Heart J. 2008;29:3022–8.
39. Dzau VJ, Sasamura H, Hein L. Heterogeneity of angiotensin synthetic pathways and receptor subtypes—physiological and pharmacological implications. J Hypertens. 1993;11:S13–8.
40. Konstam MA, Neaton JD, Dickstein K, et al., for the HEAAL Investigators. Effects of high-dose versus low-dose losartan on clinical outcomes in patients with heart failure (HEAAL study): a randomised, double-blind trial. Lancet. 2009;374:1840–8.
41. Phillips CO, Kashani A, Ko DK, Francis G, Krumholz HMK. Adverse effects of combination angiotensin II receptor blockers plus angiotensin-converting enzyme inhibitors for left ventricular dysfunction. Arch Intern Med. 2007;167:1930–6.
42. Pfeffer MA, McMurray JJ, Velazquez EJ, et al., for the Valsartan in Acute Myocardial Infarction Trial Investigators. Valsartan, captopril, or both in myocardial infarction complicated by heart failure, left ventricular dysfunction, or both [published correction appears in N Engl J Med. 2004;350:203]. N Engl J Med. 2003;349:1893–1906.
43. Hunt SA, Abraham WT, Chin MH, et al. American College of Cardiology. American Heart Association Task Force on Practice Guidelines; American College of Chest Physicians; International Society for Heart and Lung Transplantation; Heart Rhythm Society. ACC/AHA 2005 Guideline Update for the Diagnosis and Management of Chronic Heart Failure in the Adult: a report of the American College of Cardiology/American Heart Association Task Force on Practice Guidelines (Writing Committee to Update the 2001 Guidelines for the Evaluation and Management of Heart Failure): developed in collaboration with the American College of Chest Physicians and the International Society for Heart and Lung Transplantation: endorsed by the Heart Rhythm Society. Circulation 2005;112: e154–235.
44. Bakris GL, Weir MR. Angiotensin-converting enzyme inhibitor-associated elevations in serum creatinine: is this a cause for concern? Arch Intern Med. 2000;160:685–93.
45. Pitt B, Zannad F, Remme WJ, et al. The effect of spironolactone on morbidity and mortality in patients with severe heart failure. N Engl J Med. 1999;341:709–17.
46. Juurlink DN, Mamdani MM, Lee DS, et al. Rates of hyperkalemia after publication of the Randomized Aldactone Evaluation Study. N Engl J Med. 2004;351:543–51.
47. Pitt B, Remme W, Zannad F, et al. Eplerenone, a selective aldosterone blocker, in patients with left ventricular dysfunction after myocardial infarction. N Engl J Med. 2003;348:1309–21. Erratum in: N Engl J. 2003;348:2271.
48. Staessen JA, Li Y, Richart T. Oral renin inhibitors. Lancet. 2006;368:1449–56.
49. Birkenhager WH, Staessen JA. Dual inhibition of the renin system by aliskiren and valsartan. Lancet. 2007;370:195–6.
50. Seed A, Gardner R, McMurray J, et al. Neurohumoral effects of the new orally active renin inhibitor, aliskiren, in chronic heart failure. Eur J Heart Fail. 2007;9:1120–7.
51. McMurray JJV, Pitt B, Latini R, et al., for the Aliskiren Observation of Heart Failure Treatment (ALOFT) Investigators. Circ Heart Fail. 2008;1:17–24.
52. Gehr TWB, Sica DA. Hyperkalemia in congestive heart failure. Congest Heart Fail. 2001; 7:97–100.
53. Shah KB, Rao K, Sawyer R, Gottlieb SS. The adequacy of laboratory monitoring in patients treated with spironolactone for congestive heart failure. J Am Coll Cardiol. 2005;46:845–9.
54. Vanpee D, Swine CH. Elderly heart failure patients with drug-induced serious hyperkalemia. Aging. 2000;12:315–9.

Management of Heart Failure with Renal Artery Ischaemia

Andrew K. Roy and Patrick Murray

Introduction

Atherosclerotic renal artery stenosis (RAS) is commonly associated with diffuse micro- and macrovascular disease within the cardiovascular system. Patients with RAS have increased morbidity and mortality, caused by both kidney function decline and progressive cardiovascular disease. Renovascular disease can cause pulmonary oedema and worsening heart failure (HF), refractory hypertension and chronic kidney disease (CKD) with renal tubulointerstitial fibrosis. As understanding of this cardiorenal interaction evolves, it is clear that awareness and early interventions with targeted medical therapies aimed at reducing atherosclerotic burden are essential to prevent progression of renovascular disease and cardiovascular events, with further targeted revascularization playing a role in appropriately selected patients.

Definition of Renal Artery Stenosis

RAS is defined as a stenosis of the main renal artery or its proximal branches [1]. Significant RAS is defined anatomically if there is a >50% stenosis of the renal artery lumen by renal angiography, and is considered haemodynamically significant if the stenosis exceeds 70–75%. Studies using pressure wires have shown that a

Originally published in Bakris, The Kidney in Heart Failure, ISBN: 978-1-4614-3693-5

A.K. Roy (✉)
Cardiology Department, Mater Misericordiae University Hospital, Eccles St., Dublin 7, Ireland
e-mail: andyroy@live.co.uk

P. Murray
Clinical Pharmacology, University College Dublin, UCD-Mater Clinical
Research Centre, Mater Misericordiae University Hospital, Dublin, Ireland

G.L. Bakris (ed.), *Managing the Kidney when the Heart is Failing*,
DOI 10.1007/978-1-4614-3691-1_4, © Springer Science+Business Media New York 2012

pressure gradient decrease of 10% or more from the aorta to the post-stenotic distal renal artery results in exponentially increased renin release, and may be considered to represent functionally significant stenosis [2].

Aetiology of Renovascular Disease

RAS is caused by atherosclerosis in 90% of cases. Less common causes include fibromuscular dysplasia (FMD), aortorenal dissection, and collagen vascular disease. This review will focus on the management of RAS associated with the most common cause of RAS, since atherosclerotic disease is most commonly the cause of RAS associated with HF.

Epidemiology

The prevalence of significant atherosclerotic RAS is variable between populations, with estimations for the general Medicare population at 0.5%, increasing to 5.5% in patients with CKD. This is in comparison with higher risk groups, such as those undergoing screening renal artery angiography at time of cardiac catheterization, with an estimated prevalence of RAS of 30% [3]. Atherosclerotic RAS has a higher prevalence in patients with coronary artery disease than without (increased prevalence of 11–18%), and peripheral arterial disease (22–59%), reflecting the shared endothelial and atherogenic abnormalities seen in both conditions. Patients with >60% RAS and major atherosclerotic risk factors, such as diabetes and severe hypertension, have an average rate of renal artery occlusion of 7% per year [1]. Bilateral RAS has been described in up to 44% of patients with renovascular disease, with renal atrophy and ischaemic nephropathy occurring as consequence of RAS, depending on lesion severity and progression of disease.

The prevalence of renovascular disease increases with age, hypertension, aorto-iliac vascular disease, and diabetes. Macdowall et al. compared elderly patients with and without renovascular disease, demonstrating a significant age difference (mean age 80.7 years with RAS vs. 76.8 years without RAS, $p < 0.01$), as well as an increased likelihood of peripheral vascular disease in the RAS group (31% vs. 9%), and worse renal function (creatinine in RAS 201 μmol/L vs. 136 μmol/L) [4]. They showed 34% of elderly (mean age 77.5 years) HF patients had evidence of RAS >50% severity, with 13% of patients with unilateral or bilateral RAS having evidence of total renal artery occlusion.

Prognostic Outcomes for Atherosclerotic Renal Artery Stenosis

Atherosclerotic burden is one of the factors related to progression of renal dysfunction in RAS, with one study showing a 2-year dialysis-free period of 97.3% of patients with unilateral RAS, in comparison with 82.4% for bilateral RAS, and only

Fig. 1 In a cohort of patients with atherosclerotic renal artery stenosis undergoing percutaneous renal artery revascularization, heart failure is associated with increased long-term mortality ($p<0.0001$). Reprinted with permission from [6]

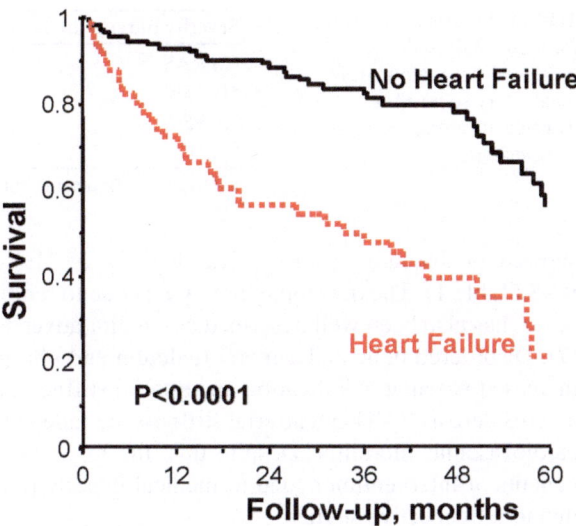

44.7% for patients with renovascular disease and solitary functioning kidney [1]. Higher cardiovascular mortality is seen in patients aged over 65 years, with end-stage renal disease due to atherosclerotic RAS, with an average life expectancy on renal replacement therapy of only 2.7 years, reflective of the overall systemic atherosclerosis burden seen in this population.

Patients with atherosclerotic RAS are at increased risk for cardiovascular events, with or without the presence of hypertension or CKD. Conlon et al. showed significantly increased rates of CKD (25% vs. 2% without RAS), peripheral arterial disease (56% vs. 13%), stroke (37% vs. 12%), and coronary artery disease (67% vs. 25%) [3]. Patients with RAS in the general Medicare population in the USA, as described by Kalra et al., experienced significantly higher adverse cardiovascular events and mortality [5].

Poor Clinical Outcomes for Atherosclerotic Renal Artery Stenosis and Heart Failure

The associations between RAS, cardiovascular morbidity, and atherosclerotic disease also influence the pathogenesis and treatment of HF, especially in older populations. Kane et al. [6] reported the presence of HF in up to one third of patients referred for revascularization of atherosclerotic RAS. The presence of HF in this subgroup was associated with a significantly increased risk of death after renal artery balloon angioplasty with stenting (Fig. 1). Estimates for mortality at 1 and 5 years for patients with HF were 23% and 73%, respectively, compared to those without HF, 8% and 35%, respectively ($p<0.001$). Follow-up studies of patients with coronary artery disease and RAS diagnosed at the time of coronary angiography

Table 1 Four-year survival
for individuals with
incidental (asymptomatic)
renal artery stenosis as
detected at cardiac
catheterization

Severity of renal artery stenosis	Four-year survival (%)
No RAS	90
50–75%	70
75–95%	68
>95%	48

Reprinted with permission from [3]

showed an absolute 4-year survival decrease of 21% compared to patients without RAS (Table 1). The development of CKD due to renovascular disease, when it does occur, has also been well described as a major adverse determinant in HF outcomes [7]. Disordered bone and mineral (calcium and phosphate) metabolism, as well as increased vascular calcification and arterial stiffness, also contribute to progressive atherosclerosis. LVH and arterial stiffness are independent risk factors for increased cardiovascular mortality. Despite this, the majority of evidence available for the benefits of intervention added to medical therapy to improve HF outcomes is limited to retrospective studies.

Pathophysiology

The pathologic effects of renovascular disease depend largely on site and severity of disease, as well as involvement of the contralateral kidney. Under normal conditions, less than 10% of renal blood flow is needed for metabolic requirements of the kidney. Significant lesions causing pressure gradients across the renal artery are thought to occur when luminal occlusion nears 70% or more, termed "critical" renal stenosis. Any variation in systemic arterial pressure can lead to significant renal hypoperfusion. Decreased renal artery perfusion pressure, detected by decreased luminal fluid chloride at the macula densa (located immediately distal to the thick ascending loop of Henle), leads to activation and up-regulation of the renin–angiotensin–aldosterone system (RAAS) by increasing renin secretion by the juxtaglomerular apparatus. This results in increased production of angiotensin II, a potent vasoconstrictor (and thus downstream aldosterone), as well as up-regulation of sodium absorption, sympathetic nerve activity and intrarenal prostaglandin concentrations.

Peripheral vascular resistance is increased, giving a similar picture to essential hypertension. In the setting of significant unilateral RAS, the normal contralateral kidney suppresses renin secretion and pressure natriuresis occurs, therefore limiting volume expansion. In the presence of abnormal contralateral renal function, or bilateral RAS, pressure natriuresis fails to occur in response to raised arterial pressures, thus making patients more susceptible to sodium and water retention, raised systemic systolic and diastolic pressures, flash pulmonary oedema, and intrarenal hypertension. Renin secretion decreases over a period of 5–10 days, thus described in the Goldblatt one-kidney, one-clip model of hypertension [8]. Medical therapies are targeted at the hypertension occurring as an important consequence of RAS, as well as the atherosclerotic process itself.

Recurrent local ischaemia occurring due to chronic renal underperfusion leads to tubulointerstitial injury and microvascular damage. Histological examinations of renal biopsies obtained during revascularization demonstrate arteriolar nephrosclerosis, and atheroembolic disease, with evidence of interstitial fibrosis [9]. These findings are the hallmarks of ischaemic nephropathy, and represent the interplay between several cellular injury pathways, in response to hypoperfusion, oxidative stress injury, and endothelial dysfunction. Pro-inflammatory cytokines, such as TNF, NFkB, endothelin-1 are involved in subsequent interstitial fibrogenesis, cortical scarring, and renal atrophy in conjunction with decreases in glomerular filtration rates. Furthermore, intrarenal atheroma and atheroembolic renal disease can also contribute to declining renal function, once 50–60% of functioning nephrons are lost. In patients with significant RAS (>60%), one of four ipsilateral kidneys demonstrates atrophy of >1 cm in length [1, 2, 8].

The Relationship of Renal Artery Stenosis to Renal Function

Impaired renal function in the setting of RAS is often called ischaemic nephropathy. While it is common in patients with atherosclerotic RAS, there is little or no correlation between the severity of stenosis and renal function [10]. The exception to this is in the setting of total occlusion of the renal artery, where compromised renal function occurs. One study estimated 27% of patients with RAS develop chronic renal failure within 6 years [8]. Progression of renovascular disease with reduction in GFR, and HF, is an independent predictor of adverse outcome. The associations between the development of left ventricular (LV) hypertrophy, anaemia due to chronic renal impairment, and the progression of HF are discussed in detail in subsequent chapters.

Cardiovascular Effects of Renal Artery Stenosis

Renovascular disease can exacerbate coronary ischaemia and systolic or diastolic ventricular function via several mechanisms. Angiotensin II, a potent vasoconstrictor, has direct effects on the myocardium, by promoting LVH and abnormalities in the extracellular cellular matrix (via multiple factors such as TNF-alpha, transforming growth factor-β (beta), IL-1), which can predispose to arrhythmias and progressive HF. It is also implicated in plaque destabilization and endothelial dysfunction, by increasing the oxidation of low-density lipoprotein cholesterol, metalloproteinase production, and lipid peroxidation. Furthermore, excess aldosterone mediated by Angiotensin II release is associated with increased collagen deposition and myocardial fibrosis. Impaired pressure natriuresis, seen in bilateral RAS and solitary kidney RAS, leads to a net increase in intravascular volume, and can precipitate acute pulmonary oedema, thereby exacerbating any underlying coronary artery disease or demand ischaemia. The increased renin release seen in unilateral RAS, with resultant increased Angiotensin II activity, can also lead to increases in LV afterload and pulmonary congestion. Other factors which may contribute to the progression of HF include increased sympathetic nerve activity, increased oxidative stress, attenuation of nitric oxide-induced endothelium-dependent vasodilatation, and up-regulation of vasopressin production [11].

In the most recent study by Kane et al. [6], examining HF outcomes from revascularization vs. medical therapy for RAS in a population with CKD, the average LV systolic function in the HF group was $47 \pm 15\%$ vs. $55 \pm 13\%$ ($p = 0.2$), demonstrating little difference in systolic function between the HF and no HF groups with RAS. The most striking feature was the presence of diastolic dysfunction both groups; however in the HF group, this was severe, with increased left atrial size (41 ± 11 mL/m^2, $p = 0.01$), and a greater prevalence of echocardiographic evidence of elevated LV filling pressures (as indicated by tissue Doppler ratio $E/e' > 15$, suggestive of increased LV volume or stiffening) 89% vs. 39%, respectively ($p < 0.0001$). This is reflective of how RAS may contribute to the pathogenesis of HF, with chronic systemic hypertension leading to diastolic dysfunction, and impaired pressure natriuresis leading to intravascular volume overload and risk of flash pulmonary oedema, as reflected by elevated LV filling pressures (Table 2).

Presentation of Renal Artery Stenosis

CKD, advanced age, and other atherosclerotic risk factors are associated with an increased prevalence of atherosclerotic renovascular disease. Renovascular hypertension can often contribute to accelerated or malignant hypertension, but is not easily distinguishable from essential hypertension. Certain well-described associations should be considered in the initial evaluation of suspected RAS; however, none has been shown to demonstrate strong predictive value (Table 3). In one study only 35% of elderly HF patients with RAS had evidence of hypertension [4]. Renovascular disease can also be asymptomatic, and essential hypertension and clinically silent RAS can co-exist, which may account for the lack of blood pressure response after intervention, seen in some studies.

Imaging for Diagnosis of Renal Artery Stenosis

Imaging studies are preferable in older patients with atherosclerotic RAS, as physiological studies, such as Captopril Scintigraphy, can often produce confounding results. Maher et al. [8] estimated the sensitivity and specificity of Captopril Scintigraphy for detection of RAS to be 85% and 72%, respectively, with limited utility in the setting of bilateral RAS. Renal artery duplex ultrasonography has a sensitivity and specificity of approximately 90–95% for detecting RAS lesions of >50%; however, this can be operator dependent. Clinically significant RAS is noted by flow aliasing on colour Doppler, and velocities across the stenosis exceeding

Table 2 Reports of renal revascularization for chronic heart failure and/or acute pulmonary oedema in the presence of renal artery stenosis

Authors and year of publication	Number of cases	Heart failure presentation	Coronary artery disease	Left ventricular systolic dysfunction	ACE inhibitor use	Renal artery stenosis degree	Intervention	CHF endpoints
Pickering et al. (1988)	11	APO	Yes 5/11	No	Yes 8/11 showed WRF[a]	7 bilateral, 2 unilateral to SFK, 2 unilateral	8 PTRA, 3 surgery	10/11 no further APO
Meissner et al. (1988)	6	CHF	Yes	Yes	Yes with WRF[a]	Severe bilateral or unilateral to SFK	4 PTRA, 1 surgery, one none	Undefined clinical improvement
Palmar et al. (1989)	1	APO	Unknown	Unknown	Yes with WRF[a]	Severe unilateral to SFK	PTRA	No further APO before discharge
Messina et al. (1992)	17	APO	Yes 11/17	Yes 6/17	Unknown	Severe bilateral	1 PTRA, 16 surgery	No APO over mean follow-up 2.4 years
Missouris et al. (1993)	2	CHF	Unknown	Yes	Yes with WRF[a]	Severe unilateral to SFK	1 PTRA, 1 surgery	Echo normalized in one, free from heart failure in other
Diamond (1993)	3	APO	Yes 1/3	No	Yes 1/3 with WRF[a]	2 severe bilateral, 1 severe unilateral to SFK	Surgery	2/3 no further APO
Weatherford et al. (1997)	5	APO	Yes 2/5	No	Unknown	1 severe bilateral, 4 severe unilateral to SFK	Surgery	No APO over mean follow-up 57 months
Ducloux et al. (1997)	1	CHF	No	Yes	Unknown	Severe bilateral	Bilateral PTRA	Undefined clinical improvement
Kwan et al. (1997)	1	APO	No	No	No	Severe bilateral	PTRA and bilateral stents	Unknown

(continued)

Table 2 (continued)

Authors and year of publication	Number of cases	Heart failure presentation	Coronary artery disease	Left ventricular systolic dysfunction	ACE inhibitor use	Renal artery stenosis degree	Intervention	CHF endpoints
Khosla et al. (1997)	28	CHF	Yes 24/28	Yes 22/28	Unknown	>70% stenosis, 8 unilateral, 20 bilateral	28 PTRA with stent	16/28 improvement in NYHA class
Planken et al. (1998)	2	APO	Yes 1/2	Yes 1/2	Yes 1/2	1 severe unilateral to SFK, 1 severe bilateral	2 PTRA	No recurrence of APO at follow-up
Farmer et al. (1999)	1	APO	Unknown	No	No	Severe unilateral stenosis of vein graft to SFK	PTRA	No APO at 2-month follow-up
Bloch et al. (1999)	25	19 APO, 6 CHF	Yes 15/25	Yes 4/25	Unknown	22 bilateral, 3 unilateral	25 PTRA and stent	18/25 no recurrence, 3 with APO, 4 with CHF at 1 year
Bhardwaj et al. (2000)	1	APO	Unknown	Yes	Unknown	Severe unilateral	PTRA	No symptoms at 1 month
Missouris et al. (2000)	9	CHF	Unknown	Unknown	Yes with WRF[a]	4 severe bilateral, 5 severe unilateral	8 PTRA, 1 surgery	Unspecified improvement
Walker et al. (2001)	1	APO	Yes	No	Yes	Severe unilateral	PTRA	No further APO

Study	n	Presentation				RAS	Intervention	Outcome
Hoieggen et al. (2001)	1	APO	Yes	Unknown	Yes with WRF[a]	Bilateral	PTRA	Unknown
Mansoor et al. (2001)	1	APO	No	Unknown	Unknown	Severe bilateral	PTRA	No SOB at 3 years
Duclos et al. (2002)	2	APO	Unknown	Unknown	Unknown	Critical RAS	PTRA and stents	Symptom free at 6 months
Gray et al. (2002)	39	CHF and APO	Unknown	Unknown	Yes 6/39	18/39 severe bilateral, 21/39 Severe unilateral to SFK	26 PTRA and stent	Reduction in hospitalization for heart failure
Basaria et al. (2002)	1	APO	Unknown	No	Unknown	Bilateral RAS	PTRA and stents	No further APO at 3-year follow-up
Aslam et al. (2003)	1	APO	Yes	No	Yes with WRF[a]	Bilateral RAS	PTRA and stent	No further APO at 6-month follow-up
Brammah et al. (2003)	1	CHF	Yes	Yes	Yes with WRF[a]	Severe unilateral, occluded contralateral	Unilateral PTRA and stent	No further CHF

SFK single functioning kidney, *NYHA* New York Heart Association, *SOB* shortness of breath
[a] Definition varies between case reports
Reprinted with permission of [11]

Table 3 Clinical features raising suspicion for the presence of renal artery disease as the cause of hypertension and CKD

1. Hypokalaemia
2. Abdominal bruit or evidence of peripheral vascular disease elsewhere (e.g., carotid arteries)
3. Hypertension lasting less than 1 year, or age of onset <30 or >55 years
4. Lack of family history of hypertension
5. Sudden and persistent worsening of previously controlled hypertension
6. Hypertension refractory to appropriate three-drug regimen (including diuretic)
7. Accelerated hypertensive retinopathy (grade III or IV)
8. Malignant hypertension (co-existent evidence of acute end-organ damage)
9. History of tobacco use
10. Acute (flash) pulmonary oedema
11. Evidence of generalized atherosclerosis obliterans
12. Asymmetry in kidney size (>1.5 cm) on imaging studies
13. Acute kidney failure with treatment with an angiotensin-converting enzyme inhibitor or angiotensin receptor blocker

2.5 m/s. Doppler measurement of renal-artery velocities can be affected by technical factors such as abdominal obesity, bowel gas, and difficulty imaging accessory renal arteries, but has the advantage of being non-invasive with no need for use of nephrotoxic contrast agents. Doppler ultrasound can also be used to calculate the renal resistive index. RAS detection rates for CTA and MRA (magnetic resonance angiography) are comparable. CT angiography (CTA) in comparison with invasive angiography has a sensitivity and specificity of up to 98% and 94%, for detecting RAS lesions >50% [12]. CTA allows for visualization of surrounding structures, especially the abdominal aorta, with the ability to quantify renal perfusion and segmental renal function. A major limitation is risk of contrast nephropathy due to the use of nephrotoxic iodinated contrast agents, thus precluding use for most renal transplant patients and those with significantly impaired renal function.

MRA has been shown to be superior to renal artery duplex in the diagnosis of main artery RAS, and is near 100% sensitive, and 89% specific compared with conventional angiography. MRA allows for the combination of anatomical and functional studies of blood flow and organ function, such as three-dimensional phase contrast MRA diffusion-weighted MR imaging. MRA has the disadvantage of being costly, sensitive to artefact (breathing, previous renal artery stenting), and has a tendency to overestimate the severity of RAS. Gadolinium, the commonest contrast agent currently in use for MRA, has been associated with risk of nephrogenic systemic fibrosis (NSF), and is contraindicated in patients with GFR < 30 mL/min. This risk is increased with the use of high-dose gadolinium in comparison with standard doses. Several combined single centre series estimate the incidence of NSF to range from 1% to 6% in patients with GFR < 30 mL/min, including dialysis patients [13].

Renal angiography using iodinated contrast media via direct percutaneous catheter injection remains the gold standard for assessment of RAS. Attempts at minimizing contrast-induced nephropathy have led to the use of other alternative agents, such as low-dose gadolinium or carbon dioxide, with modest results for image quality.

The invasive nature of renal angiography, with its associated risks, precludes its use as a screening tool.

Randomized Controlled Trials of Revascularization Vs. Medical Therapy for Renal Artery Stenosis

No trial has shown a clinically significant benefit of revascularization over medical therapy in reducing mortality, or renal function. Meta-analysis of these three trials showed only a very modest improvement in blood pressure control [14], and uncertainty about this issue remained. The commonest limitations of these studies include imprecise definitions of RAS, inclusion of patients with clinically insignificant lesions, or poorly specified medical interventions.

The DRASTIC (Dutch Renal Artery Stenosis Intervention Cooperative) trial examined renal artery revascularization vs. 2-agent antihypertensive medical therapy, in a small sample size of 106 patients. Similar to subsequent trials, RAS of >50% was considered to be appropriate for intervention, and balloon angioplasty alone was used for revascularization. The findings suggested that angioplasty had little advantage over medical therapy in terms of hypertension control, despite important flaws in relation to insufficient sample size, and classification of clinically and haemodynamically insignificant RAS lesions as suitable for intervention [15].

The STAR (Stent Placement in Patients with Atherosclerotic Renal Artery Stenosis and Impaired Renal Function) trial had similar issues with small sample size (140), and overestimation of the significance of RAS of 50–70%, particularly in the setting of unilateral disease. It found no clear differences for stent placement plus medical therapy on progression of impaired renal function [16].

To date the largest completed randomized controlled trial, ASTRAL (Angioplasty and Stenting for Renal Artery Lesions) [17], found significant risk but no clinical benefit from revascularization compared with medical management in patients with atherosclerotic RAS. The primary outcome was change in renal function over time as assessed by the mean slope of the reciprocal of creatinine. A total of 806 patients with atherosclerotic RAS at 57 centres were enrolled, over a 7-year period. This equated to two patients per centre per year. The rate of primary outcome did not differ significantly between the two groups, with no significant differences also seen in mean blood pressure or cardiovascular events or death. The rate of serious complications (23 in 230 patients, or 8%) was relatively high compared with overall combined rates in previous studies nearing only 2%. The ASTRAL trial also included many patients without clinically significant RAS (<70%), and 25% of patients had normal renal function at the onset of the trial. The issue of selection bias in the trial's design should also be considered, as many patients with high-grade lesions currently considered to be suitable for anatomic correction were not enrolled in the trial. Despite these criticisms, the ASTRAL trial is the largest trial to date, which confirms findings of previous randomized controlled trials, that, for the majority of unselected patients with RAS, intervention yields little or no significant benefits.

The most recent trial of medical therapy vs. intervention is the CORAL (Cardiovascular Outcomes in Renal Atherosclerotic Lesions) study, which is an ongoing large multicentre trial comparing the effects of angioplasty with stenting and optimal medical therapy to medical therapy alone, examining a composite of renal and cardiovascular endpoints. The CORAL trial is the first to use an optimal medical therapy treatment algorithm to protocolize and apply evidence-based guidelines for treatment of dyslipidaemias, blood pressure control, glycaemic control, smoking cessation, and use of antiplatelet agents (see Table 2).

Medical Therapy

There have been no randomized, controlled trials comparing different medical therapy regimes on outcomes in RAS. There are also no RAS specific-guidelines for optimal medical therapies, thus treatments are adapted to address the multiple aetiologies of systemic atherosclerosis. Therapeutic options are targeted at blood pressure control, via RAAS blockade using ACE inhibitor, ARB, calcium channel blockers, alpha and beta-blockers, and diuretics. Management of dyslipidaemias using current guidelines for low-density lipoprotein targets is recommended, as RAS is considered as a coronary artery disease equivalent in terms of cardiovascular risk [18, 19].

The use of RAAS antagonists may cause reduction in GFR, particularly in bilateral RAS or solitary kidney RAS. Previous studies would suggest the actual incidence of acute renal failure with RAAS antagonists is as low as 5%, and is usually reversible on cessation of the medication. In a review of 12 studies evaluating CKD progression (without RAS), the authors suggested a rise in serum creatinine of greater than 30% from baseline or hyperkalaemia, upon initiation of ACE inhibitor/ARB therapy, should prompt discontinuation of the ACE inhibitor or ARB, if occurring within 2 months of therapy initiation. These risks must be weighed up against preservation of renal function, which can occur in the contralateral kidney, positive effects on ventricular afterload in HF, and reduction of cardiac remodeling, which may occur with poorly controlled systemic hypertension. Alternative options then include progression to revascularization, or the combination of hydralazine and nitrates.

Surgical Management

Surgical approaches for renal artery revascularization include aortorenal bypass, renal artery thromboendarterectomy, and combined surgical renal artery repair with repair of concomitant aortic disease. The reported benefits of surgical revascularization for improvement of HF symptoms have been described in small registries or anecdotal reports, and are beyond the scope of this review.

Percutaneous Intervention

If RAS is clinically silent, most of the evidence suggests that intervention has no benefit. There have been no prospective trials to date showing survival benefits from renal artery intervention, despite trends shown otherwise in previous retrospective studies and registry databases.

Percutaneous renal artery revascularization using balloon angioplasty alone is recommended for RAS due to FMD where medical therapy alone is inadequate to control hypertension. Multiple single-centre studies have demonstrated the benefits of balloon angioplasty, in terms of blood pressure response, and reduction or cessation of antihypertensive medications. Predictors of success include female age <40 years at diagnosis, non-smoker, and systolic blood pressure below 160 mmHg, or hypertension duration less than 5 years [10]. However, the three multicentre trials of percutaneous balloon renal angioplasty without stenting in atherosclerotic RAS failed to demonstrate improved cardiovascular outcomes or blood pressure benefits. Renal artery stenting is superior to balloon angioplasty for atherosclerotic RAS, with calcific plaques often extending into the renal artery from the aorta, thereby affecting the ostium of the renal artery more commonly [2, 8, 10, 14]. Restenosis rates of renal arteries undergoing stent placement compared to balloon angioplasty alone (14% vs. 26–48%) are significantly lower, with ostial vessel patency rates of 57% for balloon angioplasty only vs. 88% for stent plus balloon angioplasty. Nonetheless, in this randomized study no differences were seen between the two groups in outcomes in terms of hypertension or renal function improvement [20].

Who Is Stenting Likely to Benefit?

Several studies examining the outcomes of renal artery stenting on kidney function, in patients with CKD, have shown little or no benefits. This is in part due to the limiting factors of many studies—small sample size, retrospective studies, registry reports, and single centre experiences. Zeller et al. [21] found a mean increase in creatinine of 1.1 mg/dL, in 48% of patients, with 52% of patients having only minimal (0.22 mg/dL) improvements in creatinine. Patients with evidence of cortical necrosis, significant renal atrophy, or biopsy proven interstitial fibrosis, have shown no benefits in blood pressure or renal function from intervention [22]. This lack of benefit of renal function improvement with revascularization has, to date, been replicated in larger randomized trials, such as ASTRAL, EMMA, the Scottish and Newcastle Renal Artery Stenosis Collaborative Group, and DRASTIC [12].

Table 4 Recommendations and consensus-based guidelines for renal artery revascularization [1, 2, 6, 7, 10, 24]

Intervention is *not* recommended for patients with stable renal function over 6–12 months, and whose hypertension can be controlled medically
Intervention *should be considered* in patients with bilateral RAS, or stenosis to a single functioning kidney in the following situations
(a) For patients with recurrent episodes of congestive heart failure without an obvious cardiac cause
(b) For patients demonstrating rapid decline in renal function over 3–6 months, without alternative obvious cause
(c) For patients in whom it is impossible to control hypertension with intensive medical therapy using at least three optimally dosed antihypertensives, one of which being a diuretic

Indications for Intervention (Table 4)

Effects on HF of Revascularization

Retrospective studies available have demonstrated some benefits of revascularization on surrogate HF endpoints, such as NYHA grade, and number of HF re-admissions. No study to date has demonstrated benefits in mortality in the short follow-up periods. Gray et al. did report an increase in number of patients receiving ACE inhibitors from 15% to 50%, which may have contributed to outcomes of revascularization for HF patients with RAS. In a recent study by Kane et al., balloon angioplasty with stenting was associated with significantly better HF control, with intervention subjects improving their NYHA class (42% vs. 18%; $p < 0.04$), with a lower average NYHA class (1.9 ± 0.8 vs. 2.6 ± 1, $p < 0.005$) [6]. Revascularization in the HF group was also associated with a fivefold reduction in the average number of hospitalizations, of which 80% were HF related. Further information is required, and the ASTRAL cardiac sub-study, and the CORAL trial should contribute to this.

Procedural Complications

The STAR and ASTRAL [17] trials highlight the significant effects procedural complications can have on overall outcome, despite improvements in overall technique of the procedure itself. Early complications occurring during renal revascularization procedures can include renal artery dissection, aorto-ostial plaque shift, and distal atheremboli often occurring during engagement of the ostium of the renal artery with a catheter, or during balloon inflations. The commonest late complications to occur are restenosis due to myointimal hyperplasia, and progression of aortic atheroma causing further disease. Local vascular access complications, acute renal failure, and death have also been reported. Complication rates associated with stenting range from 18% to 33% [23, 24], with restenosis rates at 1 year occurring in 11–39% [25].

Distal Protection Devices

Given the risk of atheroembolism, local vascular inflammation, and silent cholesterol emboli during revascularization, distal protection devices have increasingly been used to attempt to minimize renal injury during procedures. Estimates suggest 20–40% of patients experience worsening renal function after "unprotected" renal artery stenting. Holden et al. [26] studied 63 patients who underwent revascularization with distal protection for RAS with deteriorating renal function, and demonstrated stabilization or improvement of renal function within 6 months for 97% of patients, suggesting a protective role for distal renal artery protection. The RESIST (Prospective Randomized Study Comparing Renal Artery Stenting With or Without Distal Protection) trial demonstrated that a combination of abciximab and distal protection, rather than distal protection alone, was better able to stabilize renal function post-procedure than distal protection alone.

Conclusion

Renovascular disease and RAS should be suspected in patients with severe hypertension, hypertension associated with renal dysfunction, or unexplained diastolic HF and evidence of atherosclerosis elsewhere in the body. The evidence for revascularization is still incomplete, and optimizing medical therapy to address atherosclerotic risk factors is essential, given the high rates of associated cardiovascular mortality. RAAS blockade should be considered in all patients, according to current evidence, albeit with vigilant monitoring for hyperkalaemia and changes in renal function. Given the nature of atherosclerotic disease in RAS, statins should also be considered in all patients. Current guidelines offer retrospective and registry-based recommendations for the subgroup of RAS patients who will benefit from revascularization, and the role for revascularization in HF patients, while offering benefit in select patients, requires an appropriately designed randomized controlled trial.

References

1. Hirsch AT, Haskal ZJ, Hertzer NR, et al. ACC/AHA 2005 guidelines for the management of patients with peripheral arterial disease (lower extremity, renal, mesenteric, and abdominal aortic): a collaborative report from the American Association for Vascular Surgery/Society for Vascular Surgery, Society for Cardiovascular Angiography and Interventions, Society for Vascular Medicine and Biology, Society of Interventional Radiology, and the ACC/AHA Task Force on Practice Guidelines (Writing Committee to Develop Guidelines for the Management of Patients With Peripheral Arterial Disease). Am J Kidney Dis. 2004;43:S101–6.
2. De Bruyne B, Manoharan G, Piljs NH, et al. Assessment of renal artery stenosis severity by pressure gradient measurements. J Am Coll Cardiol. 2006;48:1851–5.

3. Conlon PJ, Little MA, Pieper K, et al. Severity of renal vascular disease predicts mortality in patients undergoing coronary angiography. Kidney Int. 2001;60:1490–7.
4. Macdowall P, Kalra PA, O'Donoghue DJ, et al. Risk of morbidity from renovascular disease in elderly patients with congestive cardiac failure. Lancet. 1998;352:13–6.
5. Kalra PA, Guo H, Kausz AT, et al. Atherosclerotic renal vascular disease in United States patients aged 67 years and older: risk factors, revascularization, and prognosis. Kidney Int. 2005;68:293–301.
6. Kane GC, Xu N, Mistrik E, et al. Renal artery revascularization improves heart failure control in patients with atherosclerotic renal artery stenosis. Nephrol Dial Transplant. 2010;25:813–20.
7. Smith GL, Lichtman JH, Bracken MB, et al. Renal impairment and outcomes in heart failure: systematic review and meta-analysis. J Am Coll Cardiol. 2006;10:1987–96.
8. Rao MV, Murray P, Yancy C. Management of heart failure with renal artery ischaemia. Heart Fail Clin. 2008;4:465–78.
9. Textor SC. Ischaemic nephropathy: where are we now? J Am Soc Nephrol. 2004;15:1974–82.
10. Dworkin LD, Cooper CJ. Renal-artery stenosis. N Eng J Med. 2009;361:1972–8.
11. de Silva R, Nikitin NP, Bhandari S, et al. Atherosclerotic renovascular disease in chronic heart failure: should we intervene? Eur Heart J. 2005;26:1596–605.
12. Coyler WR, Cooper CJ. Cardiovascular morbidity and mortality and renal artery stenosis. Prog Cardiovasc Dis. 2009;52:238–42.
13. Grobner T, Prischl FC. Gadolinium and nephrogenic systemic fibrosis. Kidney Int. 2007;72:260–4.
14. Simon J. Stenting atherosclerotic renal arteries: time to be less aggressive. Cleve Clin J Med. 2010;77:178–89.
15. van Jaarsveld BC, Krijnen P, Pieterman H, et al. The effect of balloon angioplasty on hypertension in atherosclerotic renal artery stenosis. Dutch renal Artery Stenosis Intervention cooperative Study Group. N Engl J Med. 2000;342:1007–14.
16. Bax L, Woittiez AJ, Kouweberg HJ, et al. Stent placement in patients with atherosclerotic renal artery stenosis and impaired renal function: a randomized trial. Ann Intern Med. 2009;150:840–8.
17. The ASTRAL Investigators, Wheatley K, Ives N, Gray R, et al. Revascularization versus medical therapy for renal-artery stenosis. N Engl J Med. 2009;361:1953–62.
18. Dworkin LD, Jamerson KA. The case against angioplasty and stenting of atherosclerotic renal artery stenosis. Circulation. 2007;115:271–6.
19. Cooper CJ, Murphy TP. The case for angioplasty and stenting of atherosclerotic renal artery stenosis. Circulation. 2007;115:263–70.
20. van de Ven PJ, Kaatee R, Beutler JJ, et al. Arterial stenting and balloon angioplasty in ostial atherosclerotic renovascular disease: a randomized trial. Lancet. 1999;353:282–6.
21. Zeller T, Frank U, Muller C, et al. Predictors of improved renal function after percutaneous stent-supported angioplasty of severe atherosclerotic ostial renal artery stenosis. Circulation. 2003;108:2244–9.
22. Weinrauch LA, D'Elia JA. Renal artery stenosis: "fortuitous diagnosis," problematic therapy. J Am Coll Cardiol. 2004;43:1614–6.
23. Stockx L, Wilms G, Baert AL. Prospects with renal artery stenting. Lancet. 1997;349:1115–6.
24. Dorros G, Jaff M, Mathiak L, et al. Four year follow up of Pamlaz-Schatz stent revascularization as treatment for atherosclerotic renal artery stenosis. Circulation. 1998;98:642–7.
25. Leertouwer TC, Gussenhoven EJ, Bosch JL, et al. Stent placement for renal artery stenosis: where do we stand? A meta-analysis. Radiology. 2000;216:78–85.
26. Holden A, Hill A, Jaff MR, et al. Renal artery stent revascularization with embolic protection in patients with ischaemic nephropathy. Kidney Int. 2006;70:948–55.

Combination Therapy in Hypertension Treatment

Raymond V. Oliva and George L. Bakris

Introduction

The prevalence of hypertension is increasing, with approximately one million people affected worldwide. Analysis of the National Health and Nutritional Examination Survey (NHANES) data revealed that 28.4% of the adult population in the USA have elevated blood pressures (BP) and is increasing with age as isolated systolic and combined systolic and diastolic hypertension occurring in over one-half of the people older than 65 [1–4]. Despite efforts over recent decades at diagnosing and treating hypertension, the impact on the risk of developing a stroke or a cardiovascular event is still high and is directly related to the level of blood pressure. Reducing BP is associated with significant outcomes; thus, lowering systolic BP by 10 mmHg and diastolic BP by 5 mmHg reduces the risk of stroke by 35% and that of ischemic heart disease events by 25% [5, 6].

Recent hypertension guidelines have stressed the importance of achieving BP control, the aim being to reach the goal of less than 140/90 mmHg in most patients, and even below 130/80 mmHg in chronic kidney disease patients with proteinuria [7]. For several years, the use of a single drug is the standard initial treatment for hypertension. A second agent was then added-on (add-on therapy), or the first drug replaced by another from a different therapeutic class (sequential monotherapy) whenever BP fails to normalize [8, 9]. However, these old practices fail to control the blood pressure of

Originally published in Bakris, The Kidney in Heart Failure, ISBN: 978-1-4614-3693-5

R.V. Oliva (✉)
Section of Hypertension, Department of Medicine, Philippine General Hospital,
University of the Philippines College of Medicine, Taft Avenue, Manila 1900, Philippines
e-mail: drrayms@gmail.com

G.L. Bakris
ASH Comprehensive Hypertension Center, Department of Medicine, University of Chicago
Medicine, 5841 S. Maryland Avenue, MC1027, Chicago, IL 60637, USA
e-mail: gbakris@gmail.com

G.L. Bakris (ed.), *Managing the Kidney when the Heart is Failing*,
DOI 10.1007/978-1-4614-3691-1_5, © Springer Science+Business Media New York 2012

patients, even in countries where the patients are presumed to have access to health care. A different approach and attitude is needed to optimize treatment regimens. Combining two drugs of different classes have been shown to be effective in the hypertension management, either as a single-pill combination (SPC) or co-administered as separate drugs. Halving the dose of the drugs substantially lowers the BP by approximately 20% and at the same time reduces the prevalence of the side effects [10–12].

The Need for Combination Therapy

Hypertension is a multifactorial process, making it complex to normalize systemic pressures by targeting only one mechanism. BP is determined primarily by three factors; renal sodium excretion with resultant plasma and total body volume, cardiac performance, and vascular tone. The interplay of these factors control intravascular volume, cardiac output, and systemic vascular resistance that are the determinants of blood pressure. The sympathetic nervous system and the renin–angiotensin–aldosterone system (RAAS) are also involved in adjusting these parameters on a real-time basis. Genetics, diet, and environmental factors may also influence blood pressure [13]. Thus, there is a need to target most of these processes to maximize treatment. Unfortunately, drug therapy directed at any component mentioned above evokes counter-regulatory responses that may reduce its effectiveness. For example, the use of diuretics initially reduces intravascular volume and activates RAAS, leading to water and salt retention, causing vasoconstriction. Addition of a RAAS inhibitor may attenuate this counter-regulatory response.

Limited BP reduction is seen with only one antihypertensive agent. The aggregate of available data suggests that at least 75% of hypertensive patients require combinations of two or more combinations [14] to achieve guideline BP targets, which is <140/90 mmHg. In a meta-analysis, the reduction in BP with monotherapy alone was only 9.1/5.5 mmHg, which is below the goal of BP reduction [15]. Several clinical trials have also shown that targeting BP goals to less than 140/90 mmHg is impossible with a single agent. The Anti-Hypertensive and Lipid-lowering Treatment to Prevent Heart Attack Trial (ALLHAT) showed that only 26% achieved the target BP of <140/90 mmHg with one drug [16]. The Hypertension Optimal Trial (HOT) showed that 45% of the participants needed two antihypertensive agents, while 22% needed three of more agents to lower BP to goal [17]. In the Losartan Intervention for Endpoints Trial (LIFE), more than 90% required at least two agents to lower BP <140/90 mmHg in patients with left ventricular hypertrophy [18]. At the end of the Strategies in Treatment of Hypertension Study (STRATHE), a higher percentage of patients randomized to the low-dose combination achieved target BP compared with those receiving sequential monotherapy [19].

Application of Combination Therapy in the Treatment of Hypertension

There are several advantages in the use of combination therapy, whether they are SPCs or co-administering different pills.

Efficacy

A fundamental requirement in combination therapy is that it lowers BP to a greater degree compared to monotherapy with its individual components, thus, SPCs approved in the market show evidence of greater BP reduction than the maximal dose of either agent alone. Combining two drugs may result in partial or complete additivity of their BP-lowering effects, depending on their pharmacologic properties, which may be complementary to each other [20]. Another important requirement in SPCs is the pharmacokinetic compatibility where combining two drugs may result in smooth and continuous BP reduction throughout the dosing interval. In general, combining drugs from complementary classes is approximately five times more effective in lowering BP than increasing the dose of one drug [20, 21].

Tolerability

The possibility of not only lowering BP but also counteracting the side effects of the complementary drug is a key consideration in any SPC. This is exemplified in ACE-I/CCB combination, where maximum doses of the CCB may cause bipedal edema due to arteriolar dilation, resulting in an increased pressure gradient across capillary membranes in dependent portions of the body. The RAAS blocker is thought to counteract this effect through venodilation [22, 23].

Adherence

One of the most pressing issues addressed using SPCs is the promotion of adherence by reducing pill burden and simplifying treatment regimen. In a study of ~85,000 patients from Kaiser Permanente showed that adherence was inversely related to the number of medications prescribed, the more pills the less adherent to therapy the patient becomes [20]. In a meta-analysis of nine studies comparing administration of SPCs or their separate components, the adherence rate was improved by 26% in patients receiving SPCs [24].

Cost

The only downside using these types of medication is cost, as branded medications are often expensive especially in developing countries. In the USA, it may result in significant co-pays that may affect medication adherence. Fortunately, some SPCs are already generic, like the combination of ACE-I and a thiazide diuretic, so is a combination of ACE-I and CCB [21, 23, 25]. The entry of generics makes SPCs more accessible to people, improving their adherence and eventually achieving goal BP rates.

Classes of SPCs

Ideal drug combinations should not only be more effective but also induce no more side effects than each component given alone. Commonly marketed SPCs with the generic names of their components are shown in Table 1. Some combinations are available in different dosages, although not all of them are approved in a given country.

Table 1 Drug combinations in hypertension treatment

Drug combination	Available SPCs
Preferred combination	
ACE inhibitor/diuretic	Benazepril/HCTZ
	Captopril/HCTZ
	Cilazapril/HCTZ
	Enalapril/HCTZ
	Fosinopril/HCTZ
	Lisinopril/HCTZ
	Moexipril/HCTZ
	Perindopril/indapamide
	Ramipril/HCTZ
	Ramipril/piretanide
	Quinapril/HCTZ
	Zofenopril/HCTZ
ARB/diuretic	Candesartan/HCTZ
	Eprosartan/HCTZ
	Irbesartan/HCTZ
	Losartan/HCTZ
	Olmesartan/HCTZ
	Telmisartan/HCTZ
	Valsartan/HCTZ
ACE inhibitor/CCB	Benazepril/amlodipine
	Delapril/manidipine
	Enalapril/diltiazem
	Enalapril/felodipine ER
	Enalapril/nitrendipine
	Ramipril/felodipine ER
	Trandolapril/verapamil ER
ARB/CCB	Valsartan/amlodipine
	Olmesartan/amlodipine
	Losartan/amlodipine
Acceptable combination	
Beta blocker/diuretic	Atenolol/chlorthalidone
	Bisoprolol/HCTZ
	Bopindolol/chlorthalidone
	Metoprolol/HCTZ
	Nadolol/bendroflumethiazide

(continued)

Table 1 (continued)

Drug combination	Available SPCs
	Oxprenolol/chlorthalidone
	Pindolol/clopamide
	Propanolol/HCTZ
	Propanolol ER/HCTZ
	Timolol/HCTZ
Dihydropyridine CCB/beta blocker	Atenolol/nifedipine
	Metoprolol/felodipine
CCB/diuretic	Amlodipine/HCTZ
Renin inhibitor/diuretic	Aliskiren/HCTZ
Renin inhibitor/ARB	Aliskiren/valsartan
Thiazide diuretic/potassium-sparing diuretic	HCTZ/amiloride
	HCTZ/triamterene
	HCTZ/spironolactone
	Furosemide/spironolactone
Less effective	
ACE inhibitor/ARB	
ACE inhibitor/beta blocker	
ARB/beta blocker	
CCB (nondihydropyridine)/beta blocker	
Centrally acting agent/beta blockers	

HCTZ hydrochlorothiazide, *ACE* angiotensin-converting enzyme, *ARB* angiotensin-receptor blocker, *CCB* calcium channel blocker

Renin–Angiotensin–Aldosterone Inhibitor and Diuretics

The combination of these two drugs results in additive effects. Diuretics decrease total body sodium triggering the release of renin and generation of angiotensin II. As a consequence, the maintenance of high BP becomes angiotensin II dependent. In the presence of a RAAS inhibitor, this counter-regulatory response is attenuated [26–28]. Addition of a RAAS inhibitor also improves its safety profile by ameliorating diuretic-induced hypokalemia. Furthermore, the uricosuric effect of the ARB losartan offsets the thiazide-induced hyperuricemia [29].

SPCs containing and ACE-I or ARB plus a low-dose thiazide diuretic are very well tolerated. In a study involving the use of benazepril and hydrochlorothiazide (HCTZ), the combination pill produced statistically significant reduction from baseline in sitting diastolic and systolic BP. In the benazepril/HCTZ 20/25 mg/tab group, the adjusted mean changes in sitting diastolic BP at end point were statistically significant greater than in the monotherapy treatment groups [30]. The perindopril/indapamide fixed-dose combination has also been shown to normalize BP within 6–9 months of treatment [31].

A post-hoc analysis of a controlled trial involving irbesartan and HCTZ, given separately or in fixed-dose combination showed that after 8 weeks of treatment, the combination therapy allowed the normalization of systolic BP in nearly 60% of patients [32].

Most SPCs contain HCTZ as the diuretic of choice; however, chlorthalidone is the more effective thiazide diuretic in reducing BP over 24 h [33]. It is not currently aligned with any SPC containing an ACE-I or ARB, but the combination of the new ARB azilsartan [34] plus chlorthalidone will be available in the future.

Renin–Angiotensin–Aldosterone Inhibitor and Calcium Channel Blocker

The combination of these drugs has been shown to provide benefit in prospective clinical trials. Addition of a RAAS inhibitor significantly improves the tolerability profile of a CCB. The former through their antisympathetic effects, blunt the increase in heart rate that may accompany treatment of a dihydropyridine type of CCB. They also partially neutralize the peripheral edema which is a dose-limiting effect of CCBs [35–37].

In the International Verapamil SR-Trandolapril (INVEST) trial, 22,576 hypertensive patients were assigned to Verapamil SR 240 mg/tab or atenolol 50 mg/tab. The ACE-I trandolapril was systematically added in patients with diabetes, renal impairment or heart failure. A relevant finding was that the combination of verapamil–trandolapril group attenuated the risk for developing diabetes compared with the co-administration of atenolol and HCTZ [38, 39]. Another study which highlighted the combination of an ACE-I and CCB was the Anglo-Scandinavian Cardiac Outcomes Trial (ASCOT), where the patients were taking two antihypertensive therapy, particularly amlodipine and perindopril. The combination regimen was found to be more effective than the atenolol-based therapy. The incidence of new onset diabetes was also reduced by 30% [40, 41].

A trial comparing two SPCs head-to-head as first line for treatment of hypertension was done by the Avoiding Cardiovascular Events through Combination Therapy in Patients with Systolic Hypertension (ACCOMPLISH) trial. It is a randomized, double-blind, morbidity–mortality trial in hypertensive patients involving two SPCs, benazepril/amlodipine and benazepril/HCTZ. The main finding was a relative risk reduction of 20% to the primary end point, which is a composite of fatal and nonfatal cardiovascular events, using the SPC benazepril/amlodipine [42, 43].

A fixed-dose combination containing amlodipine and valsartan has been developed. The most appropriate doses of the two components were established in a multicenter, randomized, parallel-group trial. After 16 weeks of treatment, BP control was achieved in 72.7% of patients receiving the amlodipine/valsartan 5/160 mg/tab, and in 74.8% of patients receiving the 10/160 mg/tab dose [44]. Another ARB, olmesartan, is available in combination with amlodipine, and study patients on this type of SPC achieved BP goals within 12 weeks of treatment and were safely tolerated [45, 46].

The direct renin inhibitor, aliskiren, has an available SPC with amlodipine. In the Aliskiren and the Calcium Channel Blocker Amlodipine Combination as an Initial Strategy for Hypertension Control (ACCELERATE), which is a double-blind, randomized, parallel-group, superiority trial, showed that patients given the initial combination therapy of aliskiren/amlodipine had a 6.5 mmHg greater reduction in mean systolic blood pressure than the monotherapy groups [47].

Direct Renin Inhibitor and Angiotensin-Receptor Blocker

The SPC of these two drugs produces partially additive BP reduction and is well tolerated. Aliskiren, a direct renin inhibitor, reduces plasma renin activity by at least 70% and buffers the increase in renin observed with ACE-Is and ARBs. This combination is an effective approach in lowering blood pressure as well as favorably affecting proteinuria, left ventricular mass index, and brain natriuretic peptide. A 30% additional BP response was observed in a study of the combination pill aliskiren and valsartan as compared with either monotherapy [48].

Calcium Channel Blocker and Diuretic

The combination of a diuretic and a CCB results in partially additive BP reduction. CCBs may increase renal sodium excretion, although not to the same extent as diuretics. Long-term therapy with these two medications may lead to vasodilation, given that volume depletion does not occur with the use of diuretics. In the Valsartan Antihypertensive Long-term Use Evaluation (VALUE) trial, HCTZ was added as a second step in patients randomized with amlodipine and the combination showed no favorable effect on either drug's side effect profile [49].

Thiazide and Potassium-Sparing Diuretics

Thiazide diuretics represent a valuable first-line option in the treatment of hypertension. However, electrolyte adverse effects limit the use of these drugs like hypokalemia, hypomagnesemia, hyponatremia, and hyperglycemia. These problems are dose dependent and can be prevented by using low doses of the diuretic [50–52]. The thiazide-induced hypokalemia is a potential cause of cardiac arrhythmias, thus the appeal of co-administering a thiazide diuretic with a potassium-sparing diuretic. In a double-blind trial, the fixed-dose combination of HCTZ/amiloride was found to be equally effective in preventing cardiovascular morbidity and mortality as compared to a long-acting nifedipine with comparable BP reductions [53]. Adding a spironolactone to a thiazide diuretic not only allows prevention of hypokalemia, but also a gain in natriuresis and antihypertensive efficacy [54, 55]. However, the use of potassium-sparing diuretics, alone or in combination, is contraindicated in patients with renal insufficiency because of the risk of severe hyperkalemia.

Beta Blocker and Diuretic

Beta blockers attenuate the RAAS activation that accompanies the use of thiazide diuretics, and their combination results in fully additive BP reduction. The addition of diuretics also improves the effectiveness of beta blockers in African-Americans and with patients with low renin hypertension [56]. The use of the SPC may be associated with glucose intolerance, fatigue, and sexual dysfunction.

Calcium Channel Blocker and Beta Blocker

A low-dose combination of felodipine extended release and metoprolol succinate produce BP reduction comparable to maximum doses of each agent with an incidence of edema similar to placebo [57]. The pharmacologic effects of these two drugs are complementary, and their combination results in additive effects. Beta blockers, however, should not be combined with verapamil or diltiazem because of their additive effects on heart rate and AV conduction resulting to bradycardia or heart block [23].

Dihydropyridine and Nondihydropyridine Calcium Channel Blockers

There are significant differences between these two classes of CCBs, as they have different structural characteristics, bind at different sites of voltage-dependent calcium channels, and there are differences in effect in the cardiac sino-atrial and atrioventricular nodes, myocyte contractility, and relaxation [58, 59]. A retrospective analysis of 50 patients with moderate-to-severe hypertension received maximum doses of verapamil and nifedipine. The study showed that the combination of these two drugs was effective and safe, and is beneficial in difficult-to-treat hypertension [60].

Less Effective SPCs

Angiotensin-Converting Enzyme Inhibitor and Angiotensin-Receptor Blocker

The combination of both RAAS blockers is not recommended for hypertension, providing little BP reduction as compared with monotherapy with either agent alone. In the Ongoing Telmisartan Alone and in Combination with Ramipril Global

Endpoint Trial (ONTARGET), patients receiving the combination ACE-I/ARB showed no improvement in cardiovascular endpoints despite BP reduction of 2.4/1.4 mmHg [61].

Renin–Angiotensin–Aldosterone Inhibitor and Beta Blocker

These drugs are both cardioprotective and are usually co-administered to patients with coronary heart disease or heart failure. However, when these agents are in combination, they produce little addition BP reduction. The superiority on the use of the vasodilatory beta blocker carvedilol in combination with an ACE-I lisinopril showed no significant effects on the 24-h mean diastolic BP or trough diastolic BP measurements as compared to monotherapy [62].

Beta Blocker and Centrally Acting Agent

These two classes of drugs interfere with the sympathetic nervous system. Together, these combination may result in severe bradycardia or heart block. When discontinued abruptly, patients may exhibit severe rebound hypertension. Thus, the SPC constitutes a less effective combination [63].

Three-Drug Combination Pill

A significant number of patients will need three or more antihypertensive medications to fully control BP. Triple-drug combination using an ARB, a CCB, and a diuretic has been available to increase compliance and adherence to therapy for these subsets of patients. The triple fixed-dose valsartan–amlodipine–hyprochlorothiazide has been shown to be effective and safe therapy for patients with uncontrolled hypertension [64]. A randomized, double-blind study using the combination olmesartan–amlodipine–hydrochlorothiazide was associated with BP reduction and was able to reach target goals after 12 weeks of therapy as compared to the dual combinations [65]. More studies are ongoing in the efficacy of triple combination therapy.

The Polypill

Several debates are ongoing with the advent of the polypill, or the combination of aspirin 81 mg, enalapril 2.5 mg, atorvastatin 20 mg, and HCTZ 12.5 mg for the treatment of cardiovascular risk factors [66, 67]. In a pilot trial, there was a modest reduction in blood pressure (4.5/1.6 mmHg) and LDL-cholesterol (0.46 mmol/L), and the drug was also well tolerated. The prospect of this type of SPC will help lower the risk of cardiovascular disease in poor developing countries, but the evidences are few to show its benefits [68].

Clinical Application in the Use of SPCs

The availability of these SPCs in the market makes an easier and convenient therapy for hypertension. Combination therapy will lower the pill count of patients who are already on several medications for different diseases. A patient who, for example, is diagnosed with type 2 diabetes mellitus who have concomitant hypertension and hyperlipidemia who on the average is taking four to five drugs, may benefit in reducing the pill count, increasing adherence and compliance. The administration of an SPC may also be beneficial even in stage 1 hypertension. In a meta-analysis, 92% achieved target goals after 8 weeks of therapy using combination of valsartan/HCTZ as compared to only 72% responders with monotherapy in patients with stage 1 hypertension [69, 70].

The American Society of Hypertension released a position statement regarding the use of SPCs that will serve as an aid in the prescription of these drugs. The following are their recommendations [23]:

1. Use combination therapy routinely to achieve BP targets.
2. Use only preferred or acceptable two-drug combinations (see Table 1).
3. Initiate combination therapy routinely in patients who require $\geq$20/10 mmHg BP reduction to achieve target BP.
4. Initiate combination therapy in stage 1 patients (at the physician's discretion), especially when the second agent will improve the side effect profile of initial therapy.
5. Use SPCs rather than separate individual agents in circumstances when convenience outweighs other considerations.

Conclusion

The management of hypertension treatment has been made easier by the entry of SPCs. These drugs have been shown to be efficacious, increase adherence especially in patients who are taking multiple drugs for different diseases, but have reduced side effects as compared to maximum doses of monotherapy. It is recommended that the preferred or acceptable drug combinations be administered in patients with hypertension. Triple-drug combination and the polypill show promise in the future, but will need more clinical trials to show their efficacy.

References

1. Hajjar I, Kotchen TA. Trends in prevalence, awareness, treatment, and control of hypertension in the United States, 1988–2000. JAMA. 2003;290(2):199–206.
2. Franklin SS, Jacobs MJ, Wong ND, L'Italien GJ, Lapuerta P. Predominance of isolated systolic hypertension among middle-aged and elderly US hypertensives: analysis based on National Health and Nutrition Examination Survey (NHANES) III. Hypertension. 2001;37(3):869–74.
3. Fields LE, Burt VL, Cutler JA, Hughes J, Roccella EJ, Sorlie P. The burden of adult hypertension in the United States 1999 to 2000: a rising tide. Hypertension. 2004;44(4):398–404.
4. Cutler JA, Sorlie PD, Wolz M, Thom T, Fields LE, Roccella EJ. Trends in hypertension prevalence, awareness, treatment, and control rates in United States adults between 1988–1994 and 1999–2004. Hypertension. 2008;52(5):818–27.
5. Macmahon S, Peto R, Cutler J, et al. Blood pressure, stroke, and coronary heart disease. Part 1. Prolonged differences in blood pressure: prospective observational studies corrected for the regression dilution bias. Lancet. 1990;335(8692):765–74.
6. Asia Pacific Cohort Studies Collaboration. Joint effects of systolic blood pressure and serum cholesterol on cardiovascular disease in the Asia Pacific region. Circulation. 2005;112(22): 3384–90.
7. Chobanian AV, Bakris GL, Black HR, et al. The Seventh Report of the Joint National Committee on Prevention, Detection, Evaluation, and Treatment of High Blood Pressure: the JNC 7 report. JAMA. 2003;289(19):2560–72.
8. Waeber B, Brunner HR. Low-dose combinations versus monotherapies in the treatment of hypertension. J Hypertens Suppl. 1997;15(2):S17–20.
9. Brunner HR, Menard J, Waeber B, et al. Treating the individual hypertensive patient: considerations on dose, sequential monotherapy and drug combinations. J Hypertens. 1990;8(1):3–11.
10. Khanna A, Lefkowitz L, White WB. Evaluation of recent fixed-dose combination therapies in the management of hypertension. Curr Opin Nephrol Hypertens. 2008;17(5):477–83.
11. White WB. Improving blood pressure control and clinical outcomes through initial use of combination therapy in stage 2 hypertension. Blood Press Monit. 2008;13(2):123–9.
12. Rosenthal T, Gavras I. Fixed-drug combinations as first-line treatment for hypertension. Prog Cardiovasc Dis. 2006;48(6):416–25.
13. Gradman AH, Basile JN, Carter BL, Bakris GL. Combination therapy in hypertension. J Am Soc Hypertens. 2010;4(1):42–50.
14. Kotsis V, Stabouli S, Bouldin M, Low A, Toumanidis S, Zakopoulos N. Impact of obesity on 24-hour ambulatory blood pressure and hypertension. Hypertension. 2005;45(4):602–7.
15. Law MR, Wald NJ, Morris JK, Jordan RE. Value of low dose combination treatment with blood pressure lowering drugs: analysis of 354 randomised trials. BMJ. 2003;326(7404):1427.
16. ALLHAT Officers and Coordinators for the ALLHAT Collaborative Research Group. The Antihypertensive and Lipid-Lowering Treatment to Prevent Heart Attack Trial. Major outcomes in high-risk hypertensive patients randomized to angiotensin-converting enzyme inhibitor or calcium channel blocker vs diuretic: The Antihypertensive and Lipid-Lowering Treatment to Prevent Heart Attack Trial (ALLHAT). JAMA. 2002;288(23): 2981–97.
17. Hansson L, Zanchetti A, Carruthers SG, et al. Effects of intensive blood-pressure lowering and low-dose aspirin in patients with hypertension: principal results of the Hypertension Optimal Treatment (HOT) randomised trial. HOT Study Group. Lancet. 1998;351(9118):1755–62.
18. Dahlof B, Devereux RB, Kjeldsen SE, et al. Cardiovascular morbidity and mortality in the Losartan Intervention For Endpoint reduction in hypertension study (LIFE): a randomised trial against atenolol. Lancet. 2002;359(9311):995–1003.
19. Mourad JJ, Waeber B, Zannad F, Laville M, Duru G, Andrejak M. Comparison of different therapeutic strategies in hypertension: a low-dose combination of perindopril/indapamide versus a sequential monotherapy or a stepped-care approach. J Hypertens. 2004;22(12): 2379–86.

20. Wald DS, Law M, Morris JK, Bestwick JP, Wald NJ. Combination therapy versus monotherapy in reducing blood pressure: meta-analysis on 11,000 participants from 42 trials. Am J Med. 2009;122(3):290–300.
21. Hopkins KA, Bakris GL. Fixed-dose combination and chronic kidney disease progression: which is the best? Curr Opin Nephrol Hypertens. 2010;19(5):450–5.
22. Fung V, Huang J, Brand R, Newhouse JP, Hsu J. Hypertension treatment in a medicare population: adherence and systolic blood pressure control. Clin Ther. 2007;29(5):972–84.
23. Gradman AH, Basile JN, Carter BL, et al. Combination therapy in hypertension. J Am Soc Hypertens. 2010;4(2):90–8.
24. Bangalore S, Kamalakkannan G, Parkar S, Messerli FH. Fixed-dose combinations improve medication compliance: a meta-analysis. Am J Med. 2007;120(8):713–9.
25. Yoshimura M, Kawai M. Synergistic inhibitory effect of angiotensin II receptor blocker and thiazide diuretic on the tissue renin-angiotensin-aldosterone system. J Renin Angiotensin Aldosterone Syst. 2010;11(2):124–6.
26. Chrysant SG. Using fixed-dose combination therapies to achieve blood pressure goals. Clin Drug Investig. 2008;28(11):713–34.
27. Chrysant SG, Stimpel M. Antihypertensive effectiveness of a very low fixed-dose combination of moexipril and hydrochlorothiazide. J Cardiovasc Pharmacol. 1998;31(3):384–90.
28. Lacourciere Y, Neutel JM, Schumacher H. Comparison of fixed-dose combinations of telmisartan/hydrochlorothiazide 40/12.5 mg and 80/12.5 mg and a fixed-dose combination of losartan/hydrochlorothiazide 50/12.5 mg in mild to moderate essential hypertension: pooled analysis of two multicenter, prospective, randomized, open-label, blinded-end point (PROBE) trials. Clin Ther. 2005;27(11):1795–805.
29. Dahlof B, Devereux RB, Julius S, et al. Characteristics of 9194 patients with left ventricular hypertrophy: the LIFE study. Losartan Intervention For Endpoint Reduction in Hypertension. Hypertension. 1998;32(6):989–97.
30. Chrysant SG, Fagan T, Glazer R, Kriegman A. Effects of benazepril and hydrochlorothiazide, given alone and in low- and high-dose combinations, on blood pressure in patients with hypertension. Arch Fam Med. 1996;5(1):17–24.
31. Hypertension arm of ADVANCE defines extent of renal protection using perindopril/indapamide in type 2 diabetics. Cardiovasc J Afr. 2008;19(4):226.
32. Croxtall JD, Keating GM. Irbesartan/hydrochlorothiazide: in moderate to severe hypertension. Drugs. 2008;68(10):1465–72.
33. Sica DA. Chlorthalidone—a renaissance in use? Expert Opin Pharmacother. 2009;10(13):2037–9.
34. Bakris GL, Sica D, Weber M, et al. The comparative effects of azilsartan medoxomil and olmesartan on ambulatory and clinic blood pressure. J Clin Hypertens (Greenwich). 2011;13(2): 81–8.
35. Frishman WH, Ram CV, McMahon FG, et al. Comparison of amlodipine and benazepril monotherapy to amlodipine plus benazepril in patients with systemic hypertension: a randomized, double-blind, placebo-controlled, parallel-group study. The Benazepril/Amlodipine Study Group. J Clin Pharmacol. 1995;35(11):1060–6.
36. Smith TR, Philipp T, Vaisse B, et al. Amlodipine and valsartan combined and as monotherapy in stage 2, elderly, and black hypertensive patients: subgroup analyses of 2 randomized, placebo-controlled studies. J Clin Hypertens (Greenwich). 2007;9(5):355–64.
37. Chrysant SG. Amlodipine/ARB fixed-dose combinations for the treatment of hypertension: focus on amlodipine/olmesartan combination. Drugs Today (Barc). 2008;44(6):443–53.
38. Cooper-Dehoff RM, Handberg EM, Mancia G, et al. INVEST revisited: review of findings from the International Verapamil SR-Trandolapril Study. Expert Rev Cardiovasc Ther. 2009;7(11):1329–40.
39. Cooper-Dehoff RM, Aranda Jr JM, Gaxiola E, et al. Blood pressure control and cardiovascular outcomes in high-risk Hispanic patients—findings from the International Verapamil SR/Trandolapril Study (INVEST). Am Heart J. 2006;151(5):1072–9.
40. Scheen AJ, Krzesinski JM. Fixed combination perindopril-amlodipine (Coveram) in the treatment of hypertension and coronary heart disease. Rev Med Liege. 2009;64(4):223–7.

41. Widimsky Jr J. Prevention of cardiovascular events by the antihypertensive treatment using amlodipine and perindopril in comparison with the use of atenolol and bendroflumethiazide. The ASCOT (Anglo-Scandinavian Outcomes Trail: blood pressure lowering arm) study results—multicentre, randomised, controlled trial. Landmark in the development of opinions on combination therapy in hypertension? Vnitr Lek. 2005;51(12):1394–9 [comment].

42. Jamerson KA. The first hypertension trial comparing the effects of two fixed-dose combination therapy regimens on cardiovascular events: Avoiding Cardiovascular events through Combination therapy in Patients Living with Systolic Hypertension (ACCOMPLISH). J Clin Hypertens (Greenwich). 2003;5(4 Suppl 3):29–35.

43. Kjeldsen SE, Weber M, Oparil S, Jamerson KA. Combining RAAS and calcium channel blockade: ACCOMPLISH in perspective. Blood Press. 2008;17(5–6):260–9.

44. Braun N, Ulmer HJ, Ansari A, Handrock R, Klebs S. Efficacy and safety of the single pill combination of amlodipine 10 mg plus valsartan 160 mg in hypertensive patients not controlled by amlodipine 10 mg plus olmesartan 20 mg in free combination. Curr Med Res Opin. 2009;25(2):421–30.

45. Bramlage P, Wolf WP, Fronk EM, et al. Improving quality of life in hypertension management using a fixed-dose combination of olmesartan and amlodipine in primary care. Expert Opin Pharmacother. 2010;11(17):2779–90.

46. Punzi H, Neutel JM, Kereiakes DJ, et al. Efficacy of amlodipine and olmesartan medoxomil in patients with hypertension: the AZOR Trial Evaluating Blood Pressure Reductions and Control (AZTEC) study. Ther Adv Cardiovasc Dis. 2010;4(4):209–21.

47. Brown MJ, McInnes GT, Papst CC, Zhang J, MacDonald TM. Aliskiren and the calcium channel blocker amlodipine combination as an initial treatment strategy for hypertension control (ACCELERATE): a randomised, parallel-group trial. Lancet. 2011;377(9762):312–20.

48. Yarows SA. Aliskiren/valsartan combination for the treatment of cardiovascular and renal diseases. Expert Rev Cardiovasc Ther. 2010;8(1):19–33.

49. Julius S, Weber MA, Kjeldsen SE, et al. The Valsartan Antihypertensive Long-Term Use Evaluation (VALUE) trial: outcomes in patients receiving monotherapy. Hypertension. 2006;48(3):385–91.

50. Siscovick DS, Raghunathan TE, Psaty BM, et al. Diuretic therapy for hypertension and the risk of primary cardiac arrest. N Engl J Med. 1994;330(26):1852–7.

51. Weinmann S, Glass AG, Weiss NS, Psaty BM, Siscovick DS, White E. Use of diuretics and other antihypertensive medications in relation to the risk of renal cell cancer. Am J Epidemiol. 1994;140(9):792–804.

52. Psaty BM, Smith NL, Heckbert SR, et al. Diuretic therapy, the alpha-adducin gene variant, and the risk of myocardial infarction or stroke in persons with treated hypertension. JAMA. 2002;287(13):1680–9.

53. Ismail Z, Triggs EJ, Smithurst BA, Parke W. The pharmacokinetics of amiloride-hydrochlorothiazide combination in the young and elderly. Eur J Clin Pharmacol. 1989;37(2):167–71.

54. Kithas PA, Supiano MA. Spironolactone and hydrochlorothiazide decrease vascular stiffness and blood pressure in geriatric hypertension. J Am Geriatr Soc. 2010;58(7):1327–32.

55. Wu SL, Du X, Xing AJ, et al. Impact of patient compliance on the outcomes in hypertensive patients receiving hydrochlorothiazide based combination therapy with spironolactone or captopril. Zhonghua Xin Xue Guan Bing Za Zhi. 2008;36(12):1078–82.

56. Hylander B, Danielson M, Eliasson K. Comparison of hydrochlorothiazide and slow release furosemide as adjuvant therapy to beta-blockers in the treatment of moderate hypertension. Acta Med Scand. 1987;222(2):137–42.

57. Haria M, Plosker GL, Markham A. Felodipine/metoprolol: a review of the fixed dose controlled release formulation in the management of essential hypertension. Drugs. 2000;59(1):141–57.

58. Galizzi JP, Fosset M, Lazdunski M. Properties of receptors for the Ca^{2+}-channel blocker verapamil in transverse-tubule membranes of skeletal muscle. Stereospecificity, effect of Ca^{2+} and other inorganic cations, evidence for two categories of sites and effect of nucleoside triphosphates. Eur J Biochem. 1984;144(2):211–5.

59. Galizzi JP, Fosset M, Lazdunski M. [3H] verapamil binding sites in skeletal muscle transverse tubule membranes. Biochem Biophys Res Commun. 1984;118(1):239–45.
60. Kaesemeyer WH, Carr AA, Bottini PB, Prisant LM. Verapamil and nifedipine in combination for the treatment of hypertension. J Clin Pharmacol. 1994;34(1):48–51.
61. Liebson PR, Amsterdam EA. Ongoing Telmisartan Alone and in Combination With Ramipril Global Endpoint Trial (ONTARGET): implications for reduced cardiovascular risk. Prev Cardiol. 2009;12(1):43–50.
62. Bakris GL, Iyengar M, Lukas MA, Ordronneau P, Weber MA. Effect of combining extended-release carvedilol and lisinopril in hypertension: results of the COSMOS study. J Clin Hypertens (Greenwich). 2010;12(9):678–86.
63. Gradman AH. Rationale for triple-combination therapy for management of high blood pressure. J Clin Hypertens (Greenwich). 2010;12(11):869–78.
64. Deeks ED. Amlodipine/valsartan/hydrochlorothiazide: fixed-dose combination in hypertension. Am J Cardiovasc Drugs. 2009;9(6):411–8.
65. Oparil S, Melino M, Lee J, Fernandez V, Heyrman R. Triple therapy with olmesartan medoxomil, amlodipine besylate, and hydrochlorothiazide in adult patients with hypertension: The TRINITY multicenter, randomized, double-blind, 12-week, parallel-group study. Clin Ther. 2010;32(7):1252–69.
66. Elley CR, Toop L. A polypill is the solution to the pharmacological management of cardiovascular risk. J Prim Health Care. 2009;1(3):232–6.
67. Wald DS, Wald NJ. The Polypill in the prevention of cardiovascular disease. Prev Med. 2011;52(1):16–7.
68. Majed M, Moradmand BS. A pilot double-blind randomised placebo-controlled trial of the effects of fixed-dose combination therapy ('polypill') on cardiovascular risk factors. Arch Iran Med. 2011;14(1):78–80.
69. Wagstaff AJ. Valsartan/hydrochlorothiazide: a review of its use in the management of hypertension. Drugs. 2006;66(14):1881–901.
70. Weir MR, Levy D, Crikelair N, Rocha R, Meng X, Glazer R. Time to achieve blood-pressure goal: influence of dose of valsartan monotherapy and valsartan and hydrochlorothiazide combination therapy. Am J Hypertens. 2007;20(7):807–15.

Edema Mechanisms in the Heart Failure Patient and Treatment Options

Domenic A. Sica

Introduction

The pathophysiology of sodium (Na^+) and water (H_2O) retention in heart failure (HF) is characterized by a complex interchange of hemodynamic and neurohumoral factors. Systemically perceived arterial underfilling sets into motion HF-related Na^+ and H_2O retention. The level of neurohormonal activation, the magnitude of renal vasoconstriction, and the extent to which renal perfusion pressure is reduced moderate this process. When H_2O retention exceeds that of Na^+ the end result is dilutional hyponatremia, which can present a particularly difficult treatment circumstance. Sodium and H_2O retention in HF can also moderate assorted aspects of the natriuretic response to diuretic therapy. The blunted response to diuretics in HF can have a disease-specific element; however, diuretic response is more commonly influenced by the rate and extent of diuretic absorption, the time course of tubular delivery for a diuretic and loop diuretic-related hypertrophic structural changes in the distal tubule.

Mechanisms of Edema Development

The pathobiology of progressive HF is linked with changes in multiple neurohumoral, and cellular systems; therein, there are recognizable alterations in the sympathetic nervous (SNS) and renin–angiotensin–aldosterone systems (RAAS), the vasopressin axis as well as vasodilatory/natriuretic pathways [1]. These disturbances are interpreted at the renal microcirculatory and tubular level in such a way that

Originally published in Bakris, The Kidney in Heart Failure, ISBN: 978-1-4614-3693-5

D.A. Sica (✉)
Clinical Pharmacology and Hypertension, Virginia Commonwealth University
Health System, Richmond, VA 23298-0160, USA
e-mail: dsica@mcvh-vcu.edu

G.L. Bakris (ed.), *Managing the Kidney when the Heart is Failing*,
DOI 10.1007/978-1-4614-3691-1_6, © Springer Science+Business Media New York 2012

intense Na^+ and H_2O retention follows [1]. The rich mixture of neurohumoral events that characteristically occurs in patients with HF oftentimes leads to uncertainty at the bedside as to what might be the main factor in Na^+ and H_2O retention. That being said there are three areas of particular relevance (among others) to the Na^+ and H_2O retention that epitomizes HF: level of renal function, activation of the RAAS and SNS.

Renal Function

The level of renal function is an important determinant of Na^+ and/or H_2O excretion. When the kidney is first exposed to HF signals the observed Na^+ and H_2O retention relates more primarily to factors other than a "reduced" glomerular filtration rate (GFR) per se; however, as myocardial function steadily declines in the patient with HF a gradual fixed drop in GFR emerges, which is compounded by reversible falls in GFR secondary to medication effects and/or drops in blood pressure (BP) [2–4]. Estimating renal function can be problematic in the HF patient, although serum creatinine values have often been suggested to be a reasonable gauge of renal function, in many instances "true" renal function is substantially lower than an approximation worked out from a specific serum creatinine value. Accordingly, the contribution of a reduced (or falling) GFR to Na^+ and H_2O retention can go poorly appreciated when conventional measures of renal function are used.

In the HF patient with progressive renal disease diuretics typically lose a portion of their effectiveness in that there is a GFR-dependent drop in the filtered load of Na^+. In other instances, transient changes in the GFR, promoted by systemic hemodynamic changes can delimit the natriuretic response to a loop diuretic. For example, the decrease in BP that takes place with an ACE inhibitor can lower renal perfusion pressure (and GFR) to such a degree that diuretic effect can be appreciably blunted [5]. As mentioned, changes in renal function in the HF patient can be acute and/or chronic in nature with each having a recognizable relationship to diuretic action.

Renin–Angiotensin–Aldosterone

The kidney contains various components of the RAAS; thus, angiotensin-II (Ang-II) can be both autocrine and paracrine in its renal actions. This is important in that Ang-II promotes Na^+ transport in multiple nephron segments including the: proximal tubule, cortical collecting duct, and indirectly in the inner medulla. The excess of angiotensin-II in HF [1] also has vascular/hemodynamic and cellular effects [6], which have considerable bearing (both directly and indirectly) on the renal handling of Na^+ and H_2O including: directly stimulating proximal tubular Na^+ absorption, inducing systemic vasoconstriction and increasing afterload, constricting the efferent (post-glomerular) arteriole (increases filtration fraction thereby altering the balance of hydrostatic and oncotic forces), contracting mesangial cells (diminishing glomerular filtration surface), increasing the release of aldosterone and endothelin, and by serving as a potent dipsogen (despite a typically low serum osmolality in the patient with HF) and stimulator of Na^+ appetite [7]. Of note, within organ local RAAS activation can explain the Na^+ retention, which can occasionally be seen in the absence of recognizable alterations in circulating Ang-II concentrations.

Administration of any RAAS modifying agent, particularly in those patients with a reduced systolic function form of HF, can either improve (and facilitate Na^+ excretion), or in the case of those with unstable renal hemodynamics lead to deterioration in renal function and in so doing have a worsening effect on overall Na^+ balance [8]. For example, in untreated low output forms of HF, the reduced ejection fraction reduces afferent arteriolar flow prompting local release of Ang-II, which then increases efferent arteriolar tone. This pairing of hemodynamic effects maintains sufficient glomerular hydrostatic pressure to preserve the GFR despite a low-flow state. When either an ACE inhibitor or an angiotensin receptor blocker (ARB) is administered in such a setting, the decrease in Ang-II production (or activity) will dilate the post-glomerular circulation. In combination with a reduction in systemic BP, this hemodynamic adjustment will oftentimes substantially reduce hydrostatic pressures with an ensuing fall in GFR [9].

Sympathetic Nervous System

Early in its development HF is characterized by heightened sympathetic activity [10]. Such activity adversely effects multiple organs and, in particular, the heart and kidneys. Although such neurohormonal activation is of some early benefit, helping to maintain systemic BP and perfusion to vital organs, it can become counterproductive over the long term when it goes unchecked [11]. Increases in renal sympathetic nerve activity decrease urinary excretion of Na^+ and H_2O through assorted pathways including: a heightening of tubular Na^+ reabsorption throughout multiple nephron segments, a fall in both renal blood flow (RBF) and GFR derived from renal vasoconstriction, and an increase in RAAS activity from heightened renin release [12]. Sympathetic activation can then be viewed as one of the several factors contributing to the intense renal Na^+ and H_2O retention that often develops in patients with HF [13]. In this regard, renal denervation has been shown to decrease Na^+ retention in experimental HF [12]. In addition, this process can be irregularly altered by α (alpha) and/or β (beta)-blockade; however, this remains a debated pharmacologic effect [14]. When Na^+ and H_2O handling improves with α and/or β-blockade in HF, renal hemodynamics (cardiac or directly renal related) and renal Na^+ excretory capacity (decrease in renal sympathetic nerve and/or RAAS activity) generally have improved [15]. In that regard, carvedilol may be preferable to metoprolol to prevent the development of chronic kidney disease (CKD) during β-blocker therapy for HF [16].

Renal Venous Pressure

In the setting of acute decompensated heart failure (ADHF), increased renal venous pressure may result in sufficient increases in renal interstitial pressure than renal function is worsened and/or diuretic-resistance ensues [17]. Relief of such tissue congestion/heightened pressures with strategies such as ultrafiltration may be the basis for the improvement in renal function and restoration of diuretic responsiveness in certain type of patients with HF [18]. To date, however the HF phenotype of such patients is poorly worked out.

Overview of Edema Therapy in Heart Failure

As such, multiple mechanistic-based treatments including: β-adrenergic receptor antagonism, ACE inhibition, angiotensin-receptor antagonism, and/or aldosterone-receptor antagonism are viewed as therapies that can either directly (or indirectly) influence chronic Na^+ and H_2O balance in HF [19]. Diuretic therapy and dietary Na^+ restriction are typically positioned in treatment regimens involving these therapies with well-established patterns of usage in both acute and chronic circumstances. Much debate exists as to the exact benefit afforded the HF patients managed with diuretic therapy as a component of their treatment plan enough so that in carefully selected patients diuretic therapy can be safely withdrawn and the HF managed with Na^+ restriction and neurohumoral blockade [20]. There is little dispute that diuretic therapy can in most instances treat the volume overload component of HF; however, there is simmering debate about the effect of diuretic therapy on outcomes with little meaningful data being available that show survival benefits with these drugs [21–23].

Individual Classes of Diuretics

Osmotic Diuretics

Mannitol is a polysaccharide diuretic given intravenously that is freely eliminated by glomerular filtration. Mannitol is poorly reabsorbed along the length of the nephron and thereby exerts a dose-dependent osmotic effect. This osmotic effect traps water and solutes in the tubular fluid, thus increasing Na^+ and H_2O excretion. The plasma half-life for mannitol depends on the level of renal function but usually is between 30 and 60 min, thus its diuretic properties are at best transient. Because mannitol also affects a solvent drag, it expands extracellular volume and can precipitate pulmonary edema in patients with HF; as such, it should be cautiously used in these patients if at all. Moreover, excessive mannitol administration, particularly when the GFR is reduced, can cause dilutional hyponatremia, hyperkalemia, and/

or acute renal failure. The onset of acute renal failure is dose dependent, relates to afferent arteriolar vasoconstriction, and more often than not corrects with the systemic clearance of mannitol as occurs with hemodialysis [24].

Carbonic Anhydrase Inhibitors

The administration of a carbonic anhydrase inhibitor ordinarily results in a brisk alkaline diuresis. By inhibiting carbonic anhydrase, these compounds decrease the generation of intracellular H^+, which is a prerequisite for the absorption of Na^+; therein lies their primary diuretic effect [25]. Although carbonic anhydrase inhibitors work at the proximal tubule level, where the bulk of Na^+ reabsorption occurs, their final diuretic effect is typically rather modest, being blunted by reabsorption in more distal nephron segments [26]. Acetazolamide is currently the only carbonic anhydrase inhibitor employed primarily for its diuretic action; others are used topically for treatment of glaucoma. Acetazolamide is readily absorbed and is eliminated by tubular secretion [27]. Its use is limited by its transient action and because prolonged use results in a metabolic acidosis, among other side effects. In patients receiving furosemide and spironolactone therapy, normokalemic hyperchloremic metabolic alkalosis can occur and has been linked with diuretic resistance. A short course of acetazolamide and spironolactone together with the discontinuation of furosemide has been shown to correct the metabolic alkalosis [23]. Of note, under such circumstances when furosemide is reintroduced there is an additional diuretic response; however, the basis for this restored response had not been determined [28, 29]. Acetazolamide (250–500 mg daily) can be carefully used in patients with HF who have developed metabolic alkalosis from thiazide or loop diuretic use and who cannot tolerate the volume load associated with the Cl^- repletion required for correction of the alkalemic state [30].

Thiazide Diuretics

The main site of action for thiazide-type diuretics is the early distal convoluted tubule where Na^+ and Cl^- coupled reabsorption is blocked. In addition to an effect on Na^+ excretion, thiazide diuretics also impair urinary diluting capacity (urinary concentrating ability remains intact), reduce urine calcium (Ca^{2+}) and uric acid excretion, and increase the excretion of magnesium (Mg^{2+}). The latter is particularly so with long-acting thiazide-type diuretics, such as chlorthalidone [31]. The reduction in urinary Ca^{2+} excretion with a thiazide-type diuretic is a feature that may be of some bearing to the HF patient. Loop diuretic therapy is marked by significant hypercalciuria, a transient (if not sustained) drop in serum Ca^{2+} and eventual secondary hyperparathyroidism. The latter is now felt to negatively affect cardiac structure and presumably function [32]. Hydrochlorothiazide (HCTZ) is the most widely used thiazide-type diuretic. It has a bioavailability ranging from 60% to 80%, which seems to be dose proportional. Both the rapidity and the extent of its absorption can be reduced in HF and/or renal disease and its plasma half-life correlates with level of renal function [33].

The onset of diuresis with HCTZ is fairly rapid (within 1–2 h), peaking at 3–6 h, and sometimes continuing for as long as 12 h; however, but a small fraction of the total natriuretic response occurs beyond 6-h of dosing. HCTZ is not a particularly effective diuretic in the patient with HF when given at conventional antihypertensive doses such as 12.5–25.0/mg. The magnitude of the diuretic response with HCTZ in HF has a specific ceiling, which is determined by two factors: first, the lowered GFR in HF (particularly in the later stages) reduces the filtered load of Na^+ available for excretion, and second the distal tubular site of thiazide diuretic action is one where even under the best of circumstances only a modest natriuretic response can be expected [34]. By far thiazide diuretics are most useful in HF when combined with a loop diuretic [35–37].

There is some pharmacologic heterogeneity within the thiazide-diuretic class that may have some play in the natriuretic response to these compounds. For example, metolazone is a quinazoline thiazide-type diuretic with a large volume of distribution (V_D), which prolongs its duration of action and possibly how it synergizes with a loop diuretic [37]. Metolazone absorption also is sluggish and erratic, which complicates the assessment of "diuretic-resistance" in a patient with HF; namely, the failure to respond to a diuretic regimen, which includes metolazone, is usually taken to signify a worsening of the primary volume-retaining state when it can simply be a consequence of incomplete drug absorption [34, 37].

Loop Diuretics

Loop diuretics act at the apical membrane of the thick ascending limb of the loop of Henle, where they compete with chloride (Cl^-) for binding to the $Na^+/K^+/2Cl^-$ cotransporter, thereby inhibiting both Na^+ and Cl^- reabsorption [38]. Loop diuretics also affect Na^+ reabsorption in other nephron segments but in a much more modest fashion. Loop diuretics also increase the fractional excretion of Ca^{2+}, Mg^{2+}, and potassium (K^+). Loop diuretics increase renal prostaglandin synthesis, particularly of the vasodilator prostaglandin E_2 (PGE_2) [39]. Loop diuretics shift RBF to the outer cortex of the kidney, a process likely relating to their acutely increasing angiotensin-II and PGE_2. Despite this redistribution of RBF, both total RBF and GFR are maintained after loop diuretic administration to normal subjects [40].

The available loop diuretics include bumetanide, ethacrynic acid, furosemide, and torsemide. These compounds are all highly protein bound to albumin; therefore, in order to gain luminal access (site of action), they must be secreted (as is the case for thiazide diuretics) [34, 38]. Tubular secretion of loop diuretics occurs via probenecid-sensitive organic anion transporters found in the proximal tubule. Tubular secretion of loop diuretics can be slowed by raised levels of endogenous organic acids, such as occurs in renal failure, and by nonsteroidal anti-inflammatory drugs (NSAIDs), drugs that utilize the same transporter. When NSAIDs and loop diuretics are co-administered however, there is but a slight effect on the urinary delivery of a loop diuretic [41].

Diuretic excretion rates approximate drug delivery to the medullary thick ascending limb and match up with the observed natriuretic response [34, 38, 42]. The relationship between urinary loop diuretic excretion rate and natriuretic response takes on the contour of a sigmoidal (S-shaped) curve [34, 38]. A normal dose–response relationship can be distorted (downward and rightward shifted) by various clinical conditions ranging from volume depletion ("braking phenomenon") to HF or nephrotic syndrome (disease-state alterations) to drug therapies such as NSAIDs [34, 38, 42, 43]. The latter are commonly reworked in this relationship in that inhibition of prostaglandin synthesis, particularly in HF, significantly attenuates loop diuretic effect [44]. Such a lessening of effect has been associated with a twofold increase in hospitalization rate for HF in elderly subjects treated with diuretics and NSAIDs [45].

Furosemide is the most widely used diuretic in this class; however, its use is complicated by a pattern of unpredictable absorption with an average absorption of ≈50% but a much broader bioavailability range (12–112%) [46]. The coefficient of variation for absorption varies from 25% to 43% for different furosemide products; thus, substituting one furosemide formulation for another will not regularize patient absorption (and thus response) to oral furosemide [46]. Bumetanide and even more so torsemide are more predictably absorbed than furosemide [47]. The consistency of torsemide's absorption and its longer duration of action can improve diuretic efficacy, reduce fatigue, and reduce readmissions for decompensated HF compared to patients with HF receiving chronic treatment with furosemide [48].

An essential consideration with loop diuretic use in HF is the level of renal function at which dosing occurs. Renal clearance of loop diuretics is altered in renal failure with the reduction in clearance of these drugs corresponding to the decrease in GFR. In general, among the loop diuretics furosemide's clearance is most significantly changed in renal failure given that it is both renally metabolized and cleared as the intact molecule (bumetanide and torsemide have greater degree of hepatic clearance) [49].

Potassium-Sparing Diuretics

There are two classes of K^+-sparing diuretics: competitive antagonists of aldosterone, such as spironolactone and eplerenone, and compounds—such as amiloride and triamterene—which work independent of aldosterone. Drugs in this class reduce active Na^+ absorption in the late distal tubule/collecting duct. In so doing, basolateral Na^+, K^+-ATPase activity drops off, intracellular K^+ concentration decreases, and the electrochemical gradient for K^+ is lowered; thereby, the reduction in K^+ secretion. Potassium-sparing diuretics also reduce Ca^{2+} and Mg^{2+} excretion [31, 50], which is an attribute of some potential utility in the patient with HF. Since K^+-sparing diuretics are only modestly natriuretic, their clinical utility resides more in their sparing K^+ and/or outcomes benefits in HF marked by a decreased ejection fraction [51, 52].

Spironolactone is a highly protein-bound and well-absorbed, lipid-soluble K^+-sparing compound with a 2-h half-life. The onset of action for spironolactone can be quite slow, with a peak response at times 48-h or more after the initial dose. 7α-Thiomethylspirolactone and canrenone are the two main metabolites of spironolactone that account for much of its antimineralocorticoid activity [53]. Spironolactone, unlike amiloride and triamterene, remains active (as a diuretic and antihypertensive) in advanced renal failure in that it has a basolateral site of action; thus, it does not require glomerular filtration to obtain access to its site of action.

Eplerenone is a highly selective aldosterone-receptor antagonist with much lower affinity for androgen and progesterone receptors. This receptor selectivity results in considerably less gynecomastia than occurs with spironolactone [51]. Typically, eplerenone is a very mild diuretic; thus, its antihypertensive effects arise from nondiuretic aspects of its action. It has not been studied as to its diuretic effect in HF, either given alone or administered together with a loop and/or thiazide diuretic [54].

Amiloride and triamterene are K^+-sparing diuretics that block epithelial Na^+ channels (ENaC) in the luminal membrane of the collecting duct. They are both actively secreted by cationic transporters present in the proximal tubule and have only a very modest natriuretic effect. Both drugs are sparingly used in HF even as increased expression of renal ENaC subunits may contribute to the renal Na^+ and H_2O retention observed during HF [55, 56]. These compounds may also be of some utility in that they have strong K^+ and Mg^{2+}-sparing properties [57]. Amiloride and triamterene both are extensively renally cleared and will accumulate with repetitive dosing (unlike spironolactone) in the setting of a reduced GFR. Of note, when triamterene is given together with an NSAID, acute renal failure has been reported to occur. This form of acute kidney injury may last for days beyond drug discontinuation [58].

Refractoriness to Diuretics in Heart Failure

There is a clinically relevant time course for urinary delivery at which the natriuretic response to a loop diuretic is optimized. In patients with HF, the relationship between urinary Na^+ excretion and urinary diuretic excretion rate is blunted compared with normal subjects with a downward and rightward shift of the dose–response curve. Typically, HF patients with mild-to-moderate disease generate a response that is in the order of one-fourth to one-third that which normally occurs to a loop diuretic dose. The diuretic response in patients with more severe disease is smaller yet [34, 43].

The reasons for this attenuated response to loop diuretics in HF are several: first, HF is marked by a heightened absorption of filtrate in the proximal tubule. This significantly reduces delivery of filtrate to both the TAL and distal tubule the sites for loop and thiazide diuretic activity. Therapies, which decrease proximal reabsorption, can at times improve diuretic responsiveness [34]. Second, there is a HF specific effect that attenuates diuretic activity in the TAL of the loop of Henle. A possible explanation for this is altered expression or activity of the $Na^+-K^+-2Cl^-$ transporter at the loop of Henle, a process that is modifiable by renal nerve denervation [59]. Third, aldosterone effect in the distal tubule and collecting duct places quantitative limits on how much of the filtered Na^+ load (escaping absorption in the TAL) can be excreted.

A final consideration in the attenuated response to a loop diuretic relates to the process of absorption. Both the rate of absorption and the lag time for plasma appearance of a loop diuretic increase in patients with HF, particularly when the HF is decompensated. In individual patients, as dry weight is arrived at these absorption parameters partially correct [60]. The basis for these absorptive abnormalities is unclear but may involve delayed gastric emptying, which could account for the extended lag time before absorption begins, and/or intestinal wall edema [61]. The delayed gastric emptying in HF has been suggested to have a relationship to natriuretic peptide receptor A [62].

Ultimately, these processes interactively lead to diuretic refractoriness most times irrespective of the mode of administration. One clinical outcome of this HF-related restructuring of the dose–response relationship is that the threshold for effect is appreciably increased. Failure to titrate the dose of a diuretic to this higher threshold for effect is a common error in the treatment of the patient with HF. If this circumstance goes unrecognized then unwittingly, this inappropriately low dose is repetitively given and with each succeeding dose there occurs the same minimal response. A more sensible approach is to titrate a loop diuretic dose upward until a discernible diuretic response has been established; thereafter, the frequency of daily dosing with this "correct dose" can be determined by clinical need. Diuretics that are unpredictably absorbed, such as furosemide and metolazone, are associated with a different form of resistance, which is difficulty in attaining plasma diuretic levels necessary for appropriate tubular delivery of diuretic. The loop diuretic torsemide, which is both rapidly and well absorbed, is not per se associated with this type of diuretic resistance [47, 48].

In diuretic-resistant patients, rotation of loop diuretics within a class has been conceptually advanced as another way of restoring diuretic response. Anecdotal observations suggest that patients who are otherwise refractory to orally administered furosemide can spontaneously diurese when given torsemide, bumetanide, or ethacrynic acid. However, this phenomenon has not been critically studied. It is likely when orally administered diuretics are rotated that the rate and extent of diuretic absorption would vary among class members, and a different and more efficient time course of urinary drug delivery emerge. Alternatively, when intravenous loop diuretics are rotated, "improved hemodynamics" might engender a diuresis when a patient might otherwise have been resistant to diuretic effect.

Adaptation to Diuretic Therapy

Diuretic-induced inhibition of Na^+ reabsorption in one nephron segment brings forth adaptations in other nephron segments, which not only limits a diuretic's primary actions but also is a factor implicated in side effects. Although a portion of this resistance to diuretic effect is ordinarily an expected consequence of their use, profound diuretic resistance from such adaptations can occasionally be encountered in patients with HF [63–68].

The initial dose of a loop diuretic (either intravenous or oral) typically produces a vigorous diuresis, and in most patients this results in a net negative Na^+ balance state; however, this process triggers physiologic adaptations, which preclude continued volume loss with repetitive diuretic dosing. In nonedematous patients given a thiazide or a loop diuretic, this adaptation or *braking phenomenon* emerges within days limiting net weight loss to 1–2 kg [67]. The pathophysiology of post-diuretic Na^+ retention or the so-called *braking phenomenon* is quite involved. A reduction in extracellular fluid volume is one factor that activates post-diuretic Na^+ retention, which can be ascribed to an increase in both proximal and distal tubular Na^+ absorption. It has been suggested that this heightened Na^+ reabsorption may be on the basis of increased α-stimulation and/or RAAS activation; however, administration of α-adrenergic antagonists and blockers of the RAAS do not reverse the *braking phenomenon* [63, 64].

A volume-independent component to this process has also been suggested, which may be structural in nature [65, 67]. Structural hypertrophy in the distal nephron occurs in rats receiving several-day infusions of loop diuretics. These structural changes are coupled to enhanced rates of distal nephron Na^+ and Cl^- absorption and increased secretion of K^+ and are only partially related to aldosterone [68]. These nephron adaptations may contribute to post-diuretic Na^+ retention and to diuretic tolerance in humans and possibly explain why a Na^+ avid state can persist for up to 2 weeks after discontinuation of a loop diuretic [69]. Initiation of thiazide therapy in the setting of chronic loop diuretic administration can undo the structural adaptations produced by loop diuretics [70]. This may be a consideration in the earlier initiation of combination metolazone and loop diuretic therapy in the patient with HF and an edema state that is increasingly difficult to treat [37].

Neurohumoral Response to Diuretic Therapy

Neurohumoral activation by diuretics remains an important consideration in the sustained effectiveness of diuretic therapy in HF. The neurohumoral response to a diuretic is dependent on both its route of administration and the level of drug exposure. Intravenous loop diuretics have a within minutes stimulatory effect on the RAAS at the macula densa, which is self-governing and independent of volume change and/or SNS activation. This initial neurohumoral effects with an intravenous loop diuretic even though short-lived can be of sufficient magnitude to increase afterload and therein decrease RBF. These hemodynamic changes can reduce loop diuretic effectiveness in the immediate minutes after drug administration. This sequence of events presents one possible explanation for the observation that certain diuretic treated patients respond poorly to bolus diuretic therapy, yet diurese quite effectively in response to a loop diuretic infusion [71].

A second phase response to intravenous loop diuretic administration is that of a reduction in preload and ventricular filling pressures and occurs within 10–15 min of administration and is governed by an increase in renal prostaglandin production [39]. These events offer an explanation for the symptomatic relief provided a patient with decompensated HF even before a diuretic response has occurred with a loop diuretic [72]. The next stage of neurohumoral activation occurs with excess volume removal (rate or extent) and can occur with either intravenous or oral loop diuretics. Volume removal can chronically activate the RAAS and increase circulating concentrations of both angiotensin-II and aldosterone, which, in turn, can promote Na^+ absorption in proximal and distal tubular locations, respectively, and thereby attenuate subsequent diuretic responses.

Clinical Considerations in Diuretic Dosing in Heart Failure

Diuretics are useful in the long-term management of patients with chronic stable HF who demonstrate a pattern of continuing weight gain (volume excess) despite adherence to a low Na^+ diet. They are also useful in patients who experience ADHF in which case intravenous loop diuretics are considered critical components of the treatment plan. Mild HF often responds favorably to dietary Na^+ restriction (50–100 mmol/day) and low doses of a thiazide-type diuretic. As HF worsens, the GFR also decreases and patients become less responsive to conventional doses of a thiazide-type diuretic, which usually occurs as the GFR falls below 30-mL/min. Larger and more frequent dosing of loop diuretics together with more rigorous control of dietary Na^+ intake may then be called for as HF progresses.

Because of alterations in diuretic pharmacokinetics and pharmacodynamics patients with HF often appear to be resistant to diuretics [73]. The first step in evaluating a HF patient for diuretic resistance is to assess the level of dietary Na^+ and H_2O intake. At steady state, dietary Na^+ intake can be gauged from the measurement of 24-h Na^+ excretion or on a spot urine sample shortly after administration of a diuretic. As to the latter, a fractional excretion of Na^+ in excess of 2–3% within 2–3 h of oral diuretic dosing would suggest that diuretic resistance per se is not present.

Patients ingesting a high-Na^+ diet will oftentimes overwhelm the capacity of the diuretic to produce a net diuresis and weight loss. If this is the case, a dietitian may be essential to instructing the patient as to how best to reduce daily Na^+ intake to 100 mmol/day (or less). Before labeling the patient as truly diuretic resistant, it is also important to ensure that the patient is compliant with their diuretic dosing (usually twice-a-day dosing is necessary), that the patient is not taking medication that interferes with the action of diuretics such as an NSAID, and that upright posture is not inordinately influencing response [74, 75]. In addition, particularly in those individuals with a stable pattern of HF systematic reduction and/or elimination of diuretic therapy entirely can be safely accomplished with the expected attendant benefits on renal function and neurohumoral parameters [76]. Once these factors are eliminated from consideration changes in diuretic doses, type of diuretic (thiazide or loop), or route of administration (oral versus intravenous), and/or diuretic combinations can be considered as therapeutic options.

In HF patients refractory to standard furosemide doses, high-dose therapy can prove effective. Daily doses of between 500 and 2,000 mg of intravenous furosemide were administered to 20 patients with HF and refractory edema. With this regimen, a diuresis occurred, body weight was reduced, and the HF classification improved. Similar studies have reported improved response to furosemide in refractory HF when high doses of oral furosemide were employed [77]. When moderate to severe renal impairment is present in decompensated HF, a brief trial of high-dose furosemide (or another loop diuretic) is not unreasonable. Gerlag and Van Meijel treated patients with renal insufficiency (mean GFR, 32 mL/min) and refractory HF with high-dose oral and intravenous furosemide over a 4-week period. Patients experienced a mean reduction in weight of 11.1 kg and an improvement in New York Heart Association (NYHA) classification [78]. Such high diuretic doses can be viewed as a marker of the severity of the underlying HF and therein serve as a prognostic indicator.

A loop diuretic administered as an infusion is another potential means of improving diuretic response in a patient with HF and diuretic resistance. In a randomized crossover study comparing continuous infusion versus bolus bumetanide in patients with severe renal insufficiency (mean GFR, 17 mL/min), Rudy et al. observed a greater net Na^+ excretion during continuous infusion despite comparable total 14-h drug excretion [79]. The rate of urinary bumetanide excretion remained constant when infused. With intermittent administration, peak bumetanide excretion was observed within the first 2 h and tapered thereafter. In a similar study employing furosemide, a continuous intravenous infusion of furosemide (loading dose of 30–40 mg followed by infusion at a rate of 2.5–3.3 mg/h for 48 h) was compared to an intermittent intravenous bolus administration (30–40 mg every 8 h for 48 h) in patients with NYHA class III and class IV HF [80]. A significantly greater diuresis and natriuresis was observed using continuous furosemide infusion as compared with intermittent administration and was accomplished at a lower peak furosemide concentration. When continuously infused, the pattern of furosemide delivery seemingly produced more efficient drug utilization.

A meta-analysis by Salvador et al. showed a greater diuresis and a better safety profile when loop diuretics were given as continuous infusion; however, definitive recommendations could not be made because of the small and relatively heterogeneous nature of the studies included in this meta-analysis [71]. A more definitive assessment of bolus versus infusion furosemide therapy is available from the recently completed Diuretic Optimization Strategies Evaluation (DOSE) study [81]. This trial used a 2×2 factorial design employing high- and low-dose bolus and infusion furosemide therapy and in these patients with ADHF there were not any significant differences in patients reporting of symptoms and/or renal function change whether bolus or infusion therapy was being used. Although there were several methodologic issues that confounded interpretation of this study, nonetheless its findings support the continued use of bolus loop diuretic therapy [81].

Diuretic combinations can be used in HF patients otherwise refractory to loop diuretics alone [82]. Because of structural adaptation occurring in the distal nephron with prolonged loop diuretic therapy the combination of a distal-acting diuretic and a loop diuretic is particularly effective in such patients [66, 70]. Numerous reports have demonstrated a profound diuresis (several liters daily) accompanied by clinical improvement, with the addition of metolazone to a loop diuretic (usually furosemide) in HF patients previously resistant to loop diuretic therapy alone [82]. Metolazone is particularly effective as a component of combination therapy because its duration of action is prolonged, it is lipophilic, and it remains effective in states of renal impairment [37].

Spironolactone has also been used in combination with loop diuretics and has been followed by an improvement in diuretic response in patients with advanced stage HF and a reduction in magnesium losses [83]. Above and beyond the known diuretic properties of spironolactone, it has recently been shown that, as an aldosterone-receptor antagonist, spironolactone blocks a wide range of damaging tissue-based effects attributable to aldosterone, which include augmentation of vascular and myocardial fibrosis among others [84, 85]. Accordingly, spironolactone and more recently eplerenone are increasingly advocated as adjunct therapy in HF with strong survival benefits that attends their use [51, 52, 86].

Diuretic Alternatives

Diuretic therapy remains a mainstay of treatment in the patient with either acute or chronic forms of HF. There are, however, inherent limitations to diuretic use that have prompted a search for nontraditional diuretic approaches. Vasopressin receptor antagonists have been touted as having "diuretic" properties; however, although they are "aquaretic" they have not been shown to provide significant and sustained incremental benefits on Na^+ excretion when given together with the loop diuretic furosemide [87]. Isolated ultrafiltration is increasingly employed as a substitute for aggressive diuretic therapy [88]. There is a strong physiologic rationale to such an approach and it has been shown to be both safe and efficacious when compared to patients with ADHF [88, 89]; however, questions that as of yet remain unanswered with isolated ultrafiltration include issues of timing, optimal rate and extent of fluid removal, and how best to assess when "euvolemia" has been accomplished.

Conclusions

The effective use of diuretics in HF requires considerable skill. There are multiple determinants of diuretic action in HF including basic aspects of disease-state activity that center on the heart, gastrointestinal tract, and kidneys. Diuretic absorption is a key arbiter of effect and varies markedly among the different diuretics. Treatment of the decompensated HF patient with a loop diuretic infusion is a common therapeutic strategy but has not been experimentally proven advantageous over bolus loop diuretic therapy. Diuretic resistance per se is best resolved by improving cardiac function, a process, however, that is most times easier said than done. Combination diuretic therapy can prove useful in the diuretic-resistant patient and typically entails the co-administration of a thiazide-type and loop diuretic. Isolated ultrafiltration with isotonic fluid removal is a nondiuretic strategy that is assuming more importance in the management of the patient with ADHF in that congestion can be relieved and diuretic responsiveness restored. Most importantly however, meticulous attention to the control of Na^+ intake limits the diuretic dose required for effective volume control; thereby circumventing a goodly number of the neurohumoral and electrolytes abnormalities that characterize diuretic use in HF.

References

1. Schrier RW, Abraham WT. Hormones and hemodynamics in heart failure. N Engl J Med. 1999;341: 577–85.
2. Damman K, Navis G, Voors AA, et al. Worsening renal function and prognosis in heart failure: systematic review and meta-analysis. J Card Fail. 2007;13:599–608.
3. Rea ME, Dunlap ME. Renal hemodynamics in heart failure: implications for treatment. Curr Opin Nephrol Hypertens. 2008;17:87–92.
4. Voors AA, Davison BA, Felker GM, et al. Early drop in systolic blood pressure and worsening renal function in acute heart failure: renal results of Pre-RELAX-AHF. Eur J Heart Fail. 2011;13:961–7.
5. Flapan AD, Davies E, Waugh C, et al. Acute administration of captopril lowers the natriuretic and diuretic response to a loop diuretic in patients with chronic cardiac failure. Eur Heart J. 1991;12:924–7.
6. Cat AN, Touyz RM. A new look at the renin-angiotensin system-focusing on the vascular system. Peptides. 2011;32:2141–50.
7. Geerling JC, Loewy AD. Central regulation of sodium appetite. Exp Physiol. 2008;93:177–209.
8. Good JM, Brady AJ, Noormohamed FH, et al. Effect of intense angiotensin II suppression on the diuretic response to furosemide during chronic ACE inhibition. Circulation. 1994;90:220–4.
9. Schoolwerth A, Sica DA, Ballermann BJ, Wilcox CS. Renal considerations in angiotensin converting enzyme inhibitor therapy. Circulation. 2001;104:1985–91.
10. Kaye D, Esler M. Sympathetic neuronal regulation of the heart in aging and heart failure. Cardiovasc Res. 2005;66:256–64.
11. Watson AM, Hood SG, May CN. Mechanisms of sympathetic activation in heart failure. Clin Exp Pharmacol Physiol. 2006;33:1269–74.
12. DiBona GF. Peripheral and central interactions between the renin-angiotensin system and the renal sympathetic nerves in control of renal function. Ann N Y Acad Sci. 2001;940:395–406.
13. Chen HH, Schrier RW. Pathophysiology of volume overload in acute heart failure syndromes. Am J Med. 2006;119(12 Suppl 1):S11–6.
14. Heitmann M, Davidsen U, Stokholm KH, et al. Renal and cardiac function during alpha1-beta-blockade in congestive heart failure. Scand J Clin Lab Invest. 2002;62:97–104.
15. Dupont AG. Effects of carvedilol on renal function. Eur J Clin Pharmacol. 1990;38 Suppl 2: S96–100.
16. Ito H, Nagatomo Y, Kohno T, et al. Differential effects of carvedilol and metoprolol on renal function in patients with heart failure. Circ J. 2010;74:1578–83.

17. Mullens W, Abrahams Z, Francis GS, et al. Importance of venous congestion for worsening of renal function in advanced decompensated heart failure. J Am Coll Cardiol. 2009;53:589–96.
18. Agostoni P, Marenzi G, Lauri G, et al. Sustained improvement in functional capacity after removal of body fluid with isolated ultrafiltration in chronic cardiac insufficiency: failure of furosemide to provide the same result. Am J Med. 1994;96:191–9.
19. Sica DA. Sodium and water retention in heart failure and diuretic therapy: basic mechanisms. Cleveland Clin J Med. 2006;73 Suppl 2:82–7.
20. van Kraaij DJ, Jansen RW, Sweep FC, et al. Neurohormonal effects of furosemide withdrawal in elderly heart failure patients with normal systolic function. Eur J Heart Fail. 2003;5:47–53.
21. Yilmaz MB, Gayat E, Salem R, et al. Impact of diuretic dosing on mortality in acute heart failure using a propensity-matched analysis. Eur J Heart Fail. 2011;13:1244–52.
22. Peacock WF, Costanzo MR, De Marco T, et al. ADHERE Scientific Advisory Committee and Investigators. Impact of intravenous loop diuretics on outcomes of patients hospitalized with acute decompensated heart failure: insights from the ADHERE registry. Cardiology. 2009;113:12–9.
23. Hasselblad V, Gattis SW, Shah MR, et al. Relation between dose of loop diuretics and outcomes in a heart failure population: results of the ESCAPE trial. Eur J Heart Fail. 2007;9: 1064–9.
24. Weaver A, Sica DA. Mannitol-induced acute renal failure. Nephron. 1987;45:233–5.
25. Eveloff J, Warnock DG. Renal carbonic anhydrase. In: Dirks JH, Sutton RA, editors. Diuretics: physiology, pharmacology and clinical use. Philadelphia: WB Saunders; 1986. p. 49–65.
26. Cogan MG, Maddox DA, Warnock DG, et al. Effect of acetazolamide on bicarbonate reabsorption in the proximal tubule of the rat. Am J Physiol. 1979;237:F447.
27. Kassamali R, Sica DA. Acetazolamide—a forgotten diuretic agent. Cardiol Rev. 2011;19: 276–8.
28. Khan MI. Treatment of refractory congestive heart failure and normokalemic hypochloremic alkalosis with acetazolamide and spironolactone. Can Med Assoc J. 1980;123:883–7.
29. Knauf H, Mutschler E. Sequential nephron blockade breaks resistance to diuretics in edematous states. J Cardiovasc Pharmacol. 1997;29:367–72.
30. Mazur JE, Devlin JW, Peters MJ, et al. Single versus multiple doses of acetazolamide for metabolic alkalosis in critically ill medical patients: a randomized, double-blind trial. Crit Care Med. 1999;27:1257–61.
31. Leary WP, Reyes AJ. Diuretic-induced magnesium losses. Drugs. 1984;28 Suppl 1:182–7.
32. Kamalov G, Bhattacharya SK, Weber KT. Congestive heart failure: where homeostasis begets dyshomeostasis. J Cardiovasc Pharmacol. 2010;56:320–8.
33. Beerman B, Groschinsky-Grind M. Pharmacokinetics of hydrochlorothiazide in patients with congestive heart failure. Br J Clin Pharmacol. 1979;7:579–83.
34. Sica DA, Gehr TWB. Diuretic combinations in refractory edema states: pharmacokinetic/pharmacodynamic relationships. Clin Pharmacokinet. 1996;30:229–49.
35. Rosenberg J, Gustafsson F, Galatius S, et al. Combination therapy with metolazone and loop diuretics in outpatients with refractory heart failure: an observational study and review of the literature. Cardiovasc Drugs Ther. 2005;19:301–6.
36. Dormans TP, Gerlag PG. Combination of high-dose furosemide and hydrochlorothiazide in the treatment of refractory congestive heart failure. Eur Heart J. 1996;17:1867–74.
37. Sica DA. Pharmacotherapy in congestive heart failure: metolazone and its role in edema management. Cong Heart Fail. 2003;9:100–5.
38. Shankar SS, Brater DC. Loop diuretics: from the Na-K-2Cl transporter to clinical use. Am J Physiol Renal Physiol. 2003;284:F11–21.
39. Liguori A, Casini A, Di Loreto M, et al. Loop diuretics enhance the secretion of prostacyclin in vitro, in healthy persons, and in patients with chronic heart failure. Eur J Clin Pharmacol. 1999;55:117–24.
40. Sjöström PA, Kron BG, Odlind BG. Changes in renal clearance of furosemide due to changes in renal blood flow and plasma albumin concentration. Eur J Clin Pharmacol. 1993;45:135–9.
41. Dixey JJ, Noormohamed FH, Pawa JS, et al. The influence of nonsteroidal anti-inflammatory drugs and probenecid on the renal response to and kinetics of piretanide in man. Clin Pharmacol Ther. 1988;44:531–9.

42. Brater DC. Diuretic therapy. N Engl J Med. 1998;339:387–95.
43. Brater DC. Pharmacokinetics of loop diuretics in congestive heart failure. Br Heart J. 1994;72 Suppl 2:S40–3.
44. Murphy CA, Dargie HJ. Drug-induced cardiovascular disorders. Drug Saf. 2007;30: 783–804.
45. Heerdink ER, Leufkens HG, Herings RM, et al. NSAIDs associated with increased risk of congestive heart failure in elderly patients taking diuretics. Arch Intern Med. 1998;158:1108–12.
46. Murray MD, Haag KM, Black PK, et al. Variable furosemide absorption and poor predictability of response in elderly patients. Pharmacotherapy. 1997;17:98–106.
47. Vargo DL, Kramer WG, Black PK, et al. Bioavailability, pharmacokinetics, and pharmacodynamics of torsemide and furosemide in patients with congestive heart failure. Clin Pharmacol Ther. 1995;57:601–9.
48. Murray MD, Deer MM, Ferguson JA, et al. Open-label randomized trial of torsemide compared with furosemide therapy for patients with heart failure. Am J Med. 2001;111:513–20.
49. Sica DA, Gehr TW. Diuretic use in stage 5 chronic kidney disease and end-stage renal disease. Curr Opin Nephrol Hypertens. 2003;12:483–90.
50. Maschio G, D'Angelo A, Fabris A, et al. Long-term effects of low-dose thiazide and amiloride administration in recurrent renal stone formers. Contrib Nephrol. 1985;49:108–17.
51. Pitt B, Remme W, Zannad F, et al. Eplerenone, a selective aldosterone blocker, in patients with left ventricular dysfunction after myocardial infarction. N Engl J Med. 2003;348:1309–21.
52. Zannad F, McMurray JJ, Krum H, et al. Eplerenone in patients with systolic heart failure and mild symptoms. N Engl J Med. 2011;364:11–21.
53. Gardiner P, Schrode K, Quinlan D, et al. Spironolactone metabolism: steady-state serum levels of the sulfur-containing metabolites. J Clin Pharmacol. 1989;29:342–7.
54. Reyes AJ, Leary WP, Crippa G, et al. The aldosterone antagonist and facultative diuretic eplerenone: a critical review. Eur J Intern Med. 2005;16:3–11.
55. Cheitlin MD, Byrd R, Benowitz N, et al. Amiloride improves hemodynamics in patients with chronic congestive heart failure treated with chronic digoxin and diuretics. Cardiovasc Drugs Ther. 1991;5:719–25.
56. Zheng H, Liu X, Rao US, et al. Increased renal ENaC subunits and sodium retention in rats with chronic heart failure. Am J Physiol Renal Physiol. 2011;300:F641–9.
57. Kohvakka A. Maintenance of potassium balance during long-term diuretic therapy in chronic heart failure patients with thiazide-induced hypokalemia: comparison of potassium supplementation with potassium chloride and potassium-sparing agents, amiloride and triamterene. Int J Clin Pharmacol Ther Toxicol. 1988;26:273–7.
58. Favre L, Glasson P, Vallotton MB. Reversible acute renal failure from combined triamterene and indomethacin: a study in healthy subjects. Ann Intern Med. 1982;96:317–20.
59. Torp M, Brønd L, Nielsen JB, et al. Effects of renal denervation on the NKCC2 co-transporter in the thick ascending limb of the loop of Henle in rats with congestive heart failure. Acta Physiol (Oxf). 2011. doi:10.1111/j.1748-1716.2011.02351.x [Epub ahead of print]
60. Vasko MR, Brown-Cartwright D, Knochel JP, et al. Furosemide absorption altered in decompensated congestive heart failure. Ann Intern Med. 1985;102:314–8.
61. Sandek A, Bauditz J, Swidsinski A, et al. Altered intestinal function in patients with chronic heart failure. J Am Coll Cardiol. 2007;50:1561–9.
62. Addisu A, Gower Jr WR, Serrano M, et al. Heart failure mice exhibit decreased gastric emptying and intestinal absorption. Exp Biol Med (Maywood). 2011;236:1454–60.
63. Kelly RA, Wilcox CS, Mitch WE, et al. Response of the kidney to furosemide. II. Effect of captopril on sodium balance. Kidney Int. 1983;24:233–9.
64. Wilcox CS, Guzman NJ, Mitch WE, et al. Na+ and BP homeostasis in man during furosemide: effects of prazosin and captopril. Kidney Int. 1987;31:135–41.
65. Almeshari K, Ahlstom NG, Capraro FE, et al. A volume-independent component to postdiuretic sodium retention in man. J Am Soc Nephrol. 1993;3:1878–83.
66. Ellison DH, Velazquez H, Wright FS. Adaptation of the distal convoluted tubule of the rat. Structural and functional effects of dietary salt intake and chronic diuretic infusion. J Clin Invest. 1989;83:113–26.

67. Wilcox CS, Mitch WE, Kelly RA, et al. Response of the kidney to furosemide. I. Effects of salt intake and renal compensation. J Lab Clin Med. 1983;102:450–8.
68. Abdallah JG, Schrier RW, Edelstein C, et al. Loop diuretic infusion increases thiazide-sensitive Na(+)/Cl(−)-cotransporter abundance: role of aldosterone. J Am Soc Nephrol. 2001;12: 1335–41.
69. Loon NR, Wilcox CS, Unwin RJ. Mechanism of impaired natriuretic response to furosemide during prolonged therapy. Kidney Int. 1989;36:682–9.
70. Ellison DH. The physiologic basis of diuretic synergism: its role in treating diuretic resistance. Ann Intern Med. 1991;114:886–94.
71. Salvador DR, Rey NR, Ramos GC, Punzalan FE. Continuous infusion versus bolus injection of loop diuretics in congestive heart failure. Cochrane Database Syst Rev. 2004;1:CD003178.
72. Dikshit K, Vyden JK, Forrester JS, et al. Renal and extrarenal hemodynamic effects of furosemide in congestive heart failure after acute myocardial infarction. N Engl J Med. 1973;288: 1087–90.
73. Kramer BK, Schweda F, Riegger GAJ. Diuretic treatment and diuretic resistance in heart failure. Am J Med. 1999;106:90–6.
74. Flapan AD, Davies E, Waugh C, et al. Posture determines the nature of the interaction between angiotensin converting enzyme inhibitors and loop diuretics in patients with chronic cardiac failure. Int J Cardiol. 1991;33:377–83.
75. Galiwango PJ, McReynolds A, Ivanov J, et al. Activity with ambulation attenuates diuretic responsiveness in chronic heart failure. J Card Fail. 2011;17:797–803.
76. Galve E, Malloi A, Catalan R, et al. Clinical and neurohumoral consequences of diuretic withdrawal in patients with chronic, stabilized, heart failure and systolic dysfunction. Eur J Heart Fail. 2005;7:892–8.
77. Marangoni E, Oddone A, Surian M, et al. Effect of high-dose furosemide in refractory congestive heart failure. Angiology. 1990;41:862–8.
78. Gerlag PG, van Meijel JJ. High-dose furosemide in the treatment of refractory congestive heart failure. Arch Intern Med. 1988;148:286–91.
79. Rudy DW, Voelker JR, Greene PK, et al. Loop diuretics for chronic renal insufficiency: a continuous infusion is more efficacious than bolus therapy. Ann Intern Med. 1991;115:360–6.
80. Lahav M, Regev A, Ra'anani P, et al. Intermittent administration of furosemide vs. continuous infusion preceded by a loading dose for congestive heart failure. Chest. 1992;102:725–31.
81. Felker GM, Lee KL, Bull DA, et al. Diuretic strategies in patients with acute decompensated heart failure. N Engl J Med. 2011;364:797–805.
82. Jentzer JC, DeWald TA, Hernandez AF. Combination of loop diuretics with thiazide-type diuretics in heart failure. J Am Coll Cardiol. 2010;56:1527–34.
83. Barr CS, Lang CC, Hanson J, et al. Effects of adding spironolactone to an angiotensin-converting enzyme inhibitor in chronic congestive heart failure secondary to coronary artery disease. Am J Cardiol. 1995;76:1259–65.
84. Farquharson CAJ, Struthers AD. Spironolactone increases nitric oxide bioactivity, improves endothelial vasodilator dysfunction and suppresses vascular angiotensin I/angiotensin II conversion in patients with chronic heart failure. Circulation. 2000;101:594–7.
85. Weber KT. Aldosterone in congestive heart failure. N Engl J Med. 2001;345:1689–97.
86. Pitt B, Zannad F, Rime WJ, et al. The effect of spironolactone on morbidity and mortality in patients with severe heart failure. N Engl J Med. 1999;341:709–17.
87. Udelson JE, Bilsker M, Hauptman PJ, Sequeira R, Thomas I, O'Brien T, et al. A multicenter, randomized, double-blind, placebo-controlled study of tolvaptan monotherapy compared to furosemide and the combination of tolvaptan and furosemide in patients with heart failure and systolic dysfunction. J Card Fail. 2011;17:973–81.
88. Costanzo MR, Jessup M. Treatment of congestion in heart failure with diuretics and extracorporeal therapies: effects on symptoms, renal function and prognosis. Heart Fail Rev. 2011 [Epub ahead of print]
89. Cpstanzo MR, Guglin ME, Saltzverg MT, et al. Ultrafiltration versus intravenous diuretics for patients hospitalized for acute decompensated heart failure. J Am Coll Cardiol. 2007; 49:675–83.

Ultrafiltration and Heart Failure

Paul Chacko, Donald Kikta Jr., and William T. Abraham

Introduction

Acute decompensated heart failure (ADHF) is a clinical syndrome that is increasingly prevalent given the advances in cardiovascular disease management that has enabled reduction of fatal outcomes from acute coronary syndromes. Hospital discharges due to heart failure (HF) increased by 26% to 1,106,000 between 1996 and 2006, with a projected cost of $39.2 billion toward direct and indirect expense related to HF for 2010 [1]. Data from the HF registries indicate that symptoms related to congestion are the main reason for hospitalization and yet many patients are discharged prematurely with persistent signs and symptoms related to congestion [2, 3]. Diuretics have been the mainstay of treatment in offering symptomatic relief; however, they are fraught with adverse effects such as electrolyte abnormalities and worsening renal function, which in itself increases the mortality risk [4]. In this challenging scenario where adequate diuresis is not achievable, mechanical strategies such as ultrafiltration (UF) to remove excess fluid have been demonstrated to be an effective approach.

Originally published in Bakris, The Kidney in Heart Failure, ISBN: 978-1-4614-3693-5

P. Chacko • D. Kikta Jr.
Cardiology Division, Internal Medicine Department,
The Ohio State University Medical Center, Columbus, OH, USA

W.T. Abraham (✉)
Ohio State University Medical Center, 473 West 12th Avenue,
Room 110P, Columbus, OH 43210-1252, USA
e-mail: William.Abraham@osumc.edu; judy.hawksworth@osumc.edu

G.L. Bakris (ed.), *Managing the Kidney when the Heart is Failing*,
DOI 10.1007/978-1-4614-3691-1_7, © Springer Science+Business Media New York 2012

ADHF: An Overview

Data from the well-established HF registries have enabled a better understanding about the clinical profile of patients presenting with ADHF [2, 5, 6]. The ADHERE registry offers the largest cohort of patients and sheds light on the typical characteristics of patients with ADHF. Most patients who present with ADHF have a worsening of their chronic HF, rather than truly acute HF with less than 25% presenting with new onset HF. Low blood pressure [systolic blood pressure (SBP) <90 mmHg] or cardiogenic shock was observed in only 10% while a majority presented with elevated SBP [2]. Symptoms and signs of congestion were the predominant reasons for admission. Such clinical congestion is preceded by hemodynamic congestion with an increase in pulmonary capillary wedge pressure (PCWP) along with myocardial ischemia, worsening neurohormonal activation, and often worsening renal dysfunction. An estimated 37% of patients who reportedly state improvement at discharge tend to be symptomatic at the time of discharge [7]. Although the in-hospital mortality ranged between 3% and 4%, this increased markedly to 10% during a 2–3 months period. The readmission rates were alarmingly high at 25% during the same duration [6]. Varying readmission rates ranging from 13% to 25% have been noted through other published data [8]. Alleviating symptoms such as dyspnea by reducing congestion is the target of inpatient treatment with addition of other agents to reduce morbidity and mortality as the patient improves.

ADHF: Pathophysiology of Hypervolemia

The cause of hospitalization for ADHF has been attributed to symptoms that arise from congestion, whether systemic or pulmonary in nature. Irrespective of the cause, increased left ventricular diastolic pressure ensues resulting in elevated PCWP, which is relayed on to the pulmonary artery as well as the right chambers of the heart. The above-mentioned hemodynamic alterations induce changes in myocardial geometry to a spherical shape with ineffective torsional contraction and mitral insufficiency.

Increase in cardiac filling pressures, reduced cardiac output, peripheral vasoconstriction, impairment in natriuresis and diuresis are the key ingredients to cause volume overload. It is the arterial circulation (comprising 15% of the total blood volume) that maintains the cardiorenal equilibrium. The arterial under filling sets off a neurohormonal cascade that involves the stimulation of sympathetic nerves, activation of renin–angiotensin–aldosterone system (RAAS) and the nonosmotic release of arginine vasopressin (AVP). The pathway depicting these events is illustrated in the accompanying figure (Fig. 1).

Due to the underlying adrenergic stimulation and increase in angiotensin II levels, there is amplified sodium reabsorption in the proximal tubule resulting in a low sodium load detection at the distal aspect of nephron and collecting duct, which in turn enables aldosterone activity. The adrenergic activity also facilitates aldosterone

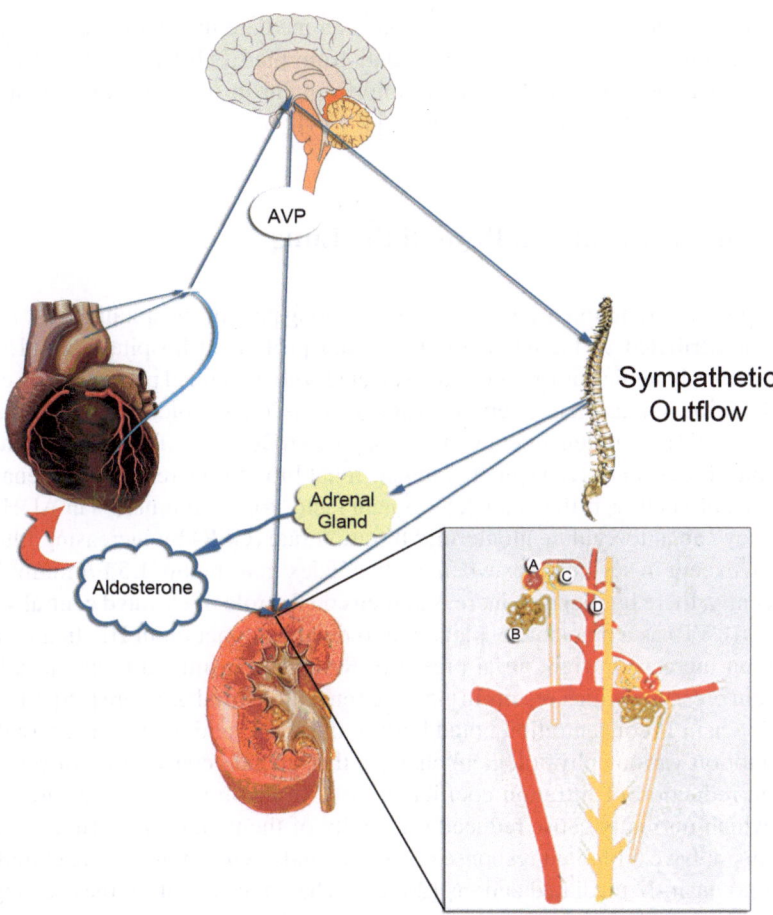

Fig. 1 Pathophysiology of hypervolemia. Decreased intravascular filling is identified by the baroreceptors in the cardiac and vessel walls (aortic and carotid arch) and stimulates the cardio-regulatory center in the brain via glossopharyngeal and vagus nerve. This generates a dual response. (1) Nonosmotic release of arginine vasopressine (AVP) which enables the aquaporin channels in collecting duct (D) to absorb more water. (2) Sympathetic outflow tract is stimulated which results in the numerous changes. Beta stimulation via renal nerves causes renin stimulation which eventually produces angiotensin II (AT II). AT II is a potent vasoconstrictor, besides acting at the glomerular level (A) causes formation of aldosterone from the adrenals and act on the thirst center in the brain to consume water as well as cause ADH release. AT II also enables reabsorption of sodium and water at the proximal convoluted tubule (B). Aldosterone facilitates the reabsorption of sodium and water from the distal convoluted tubule (C) and collecting duct (D) while ADH facilitates water reabsorption from distal part of nephron

secretion by its direct effect on the adrenal cortex. Meanwhile, the nonosmotic release of AVP cause induction of aquaporin water channels, through which avid free water reabsorption occurs [9, 10]. The end result is a hypervolemic state to preserve the intravascular compartment; with or without concomitant hyponatremia, achieved at the expense of neurohormones. It is now understood through animal models that angiotensisn II and aldosterone can mediate myocardial apoptosis and fibrosis leading to remodeling [11, 12]. Data from the EPHESUS and RALES trial support this hypothesis by the notable improvement in mortality of patients who were treated with aldosterone antagonists [13, 14].

Congestion: A Concern Beyond the Lung

Worsening renal function, a common finding among patients hospitalized for ADHF, has been attributed to increased mortality and prolonged hospital stay [15, 16]. Altered hemodynamic outflow is often associated with poor renal perfusion that causes renal function impairment. Certain drugs such as nonsteroidal antiinflammatory drugs (NSAID), angiotensin-converting enzyme (ACE) inhibitors, and angiotensin II receptor blockers (ARB) can also impair renal blood flow resulting in renal failure. Renal blood flow is the main determinant factor for renal function in ADHF and the kidney can autoregulate glomerular filtration rate (GFR) by increasing filtration fraction, except in severe cases when cardiac index goes below 1.5 L/min/m^2 [17].

Recently, there has been an increased focus on the role of elevated central venous pressure (CVP) as a plausible explanation to renal dysfunction in HF. In a systemic circuit, an increase in right atrial pressure (RAP) is transmitted to an elevation in renal vein pressure, which results in elevated renal interstitial pressure [18]. Increases in angiotensin II concentration noted both in intrarenal and in systemic circulation set in motion various physiological changes that include constriction of renal vessels and reduction of filtration coefficient [19]. In addition, atrial natriuretic peptides, which normally cause reduced sensitivity of the tubulo-glomerular feedback mechanism, have a blunted response due to the underlying sympathetic stimulation and angiotensin-II-mediated actions [20, 21]. The net effect of all these changes is a decrease in GFR, which can occur independent of cardiac output.

In an animal model, incremental increase in CVP was shown to cause reduction of GFR when renal perfusion was maintained [22]. This reduction of GFR and sodium excretion was reversed when venous pressure was relieved. In other studies, higher RAP was observed to be associated with increased mortality, irrespective of the left ventricular ejection fraction or end-diastolic diameter [23, 24]. In a more recent study, Damman et al. established an inverse relationship between RAP and GFR, independent of renal blood flow. This effect was even more pronounced when renal blood flow is reduced [25]. In a subsequent study, the very same group demonstrated a biphasic relationship between CVP and GFR, with a more deleterious effect in those with high cardiac index (Fig. 2) [26]. The graph suggests that regardless of the cardiac index, renal function is significantly compromised when there is increasing hypervolemia.

Data from the Evaluation Study of Congestive Heart Failure and Pulmonary Artery Catheterization Effectiveness (ESCAPE) trial demonstrated a lower risk of renal failure in patients with ADHF when RAP or pulmonary capillary wedge pressure (PCWP) was targeted with the aid of a pulmonary artery (or Swan–Ganz)

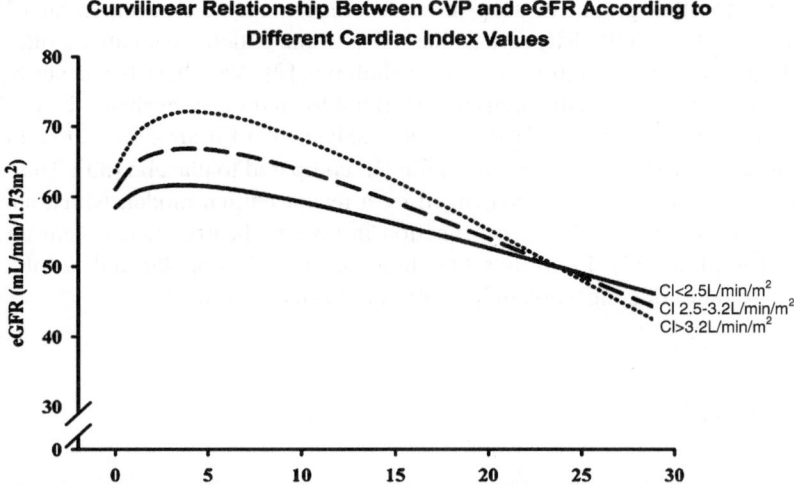

Fig. 2 Curvilinear relationship between CVP and eGFR according to different cardiac index values. From [26]. Reprinted with kind permission from Elsevier

catheter, in comparison with those who were treated based on clinical assessment alone [27]. In a subanalysis of this trial, no improvement in renal function was noted in patients who experienced a catheter-guided enhancement of cardiac index, which suggests an etiology besides forward flow as a potential cause for renal impairment [28]. This was also supported by Mullens et al. who observed that in hospitalized patients with ADHF, elevated CVP was associated with worsening renal function, when other factors such as SBP, cardiac index, PCWP, and GFR were held constant. The occurrence of renal impairment was lower in patients whose CVP values were less than 8 mmHg [29]. Hence, it is reasonable to consider that in addition to improving renal blood flow, targeting venous congestion would also help in improving GFR, and thus reduce postdischarge mortality and rehospitalization rates associated with renal dysfunction.

Relieving Congestion: Loop Diuretics, Old is Still Gold?

Diuretics have been the mainstay of treatment for congestive HF and offer symptomatic relief, irrespective of the etiology. Diuretics have demonstrated the ability to do so by increasing urinary sodium excretion and thereby alleviating the physical signs related to fluid retention [30, 31]. The efficacy to reduce pulmonary congestion and dyspnea with improvement in hemodynamics is well established among the loop diuretics [32]. There is a reduction of PCWP in the immediate setting due to the venodilatory property but the ensuing natriuresis enables reduction of ECF volume and improvement in hypoxia. They are fast acting and superior in efficacy compared to other groups of drugs used to treat HF. Acute Decompensated Heart Failure Registry (ADHERE) reveals that 88% of the patients who are admitted for ADHF are treated with intravenous loop diuretics [2]. Yet, there has never been a large-scale randomized clinical trial performed to rigorously evaluate their role in therapeutic application for ADHF. A meta-analysis of 14 trials showed that diuretics reduced the risk of death or worsening HF compared to placebo [33]. This well-established notion has been challenged by a recent animal model, which showed progression of left ventricular dysfunction in porcine hearts, which were infused with furosemide [34]. Loop diuretics, however, remain popular and are the first choices in relief of congestion unless contraindicated otherwise.

Loop Diuretics

The therapeutic effect offered by loop diuretics is via inhibition of Na–K–2Cl co-transporter at the apical (luminal) membrane of thick part of the ascending loop of Henle. These drugs are rapidly but incompletely absorbed from the gastrointestinal tract, but being protein bound, and are filtrated in limited amounts into the glomerular lumen. However, the active secretion of the compound at the proximal convoluted tubule (PCT) determines the concentration of the drug that is made available at the site of its action (loop of Henle). In renal insufficiency, this secretion is further impaired due to competitive inhibition from the accumulated organic anions for the receptor sites of organic anion transporter.

Analyzing the dose–response curve of these drugs sheds light on few important aspects about the pharmacodynamic property (Fig. 3). The sigmoid curve pattern enables us to understand that there is a threshold level, below which there is no response to the drug (Fig. 3a). Also, the plateau at the peak suggests a "ceiling effect" above which increasing the dose does not produce excessive diuresis [35]. Since the delivery of the diuretic into the tubular lumen is compromised when creatinine clearance is low, higher doses are required to maintain the same diuretic response. Hence, a shift of the sigmoidal curve to the right is noted in renal insufficiency (Fig. 3b). But in congestive HF, the curve is shifted downward and to the right, requiring a significantly higher dose but eliciting a weaker diuretic response (Fig. 3c).

Given these challenges, in clinical practice, the recommended dose to initiate diuresis is to start with a moderate dose (such as twice the outpatient oral dose or equivalent as noted in Table 1) and double it if the response in not adequate. The limiting aspect to giving higher doses is the occurrence of ototoxicity, which is often reversible in adults. There is a wide range in what is considered to be a tolerable diuretic regimen, given the variability noted from different studies undertaken to determine toxicity [36]. In general, lowest diuretic dose that produces maximal response must not be exceeded. However, the positive attributes meet limitations due to the pharmacodynamic properties of the drug.

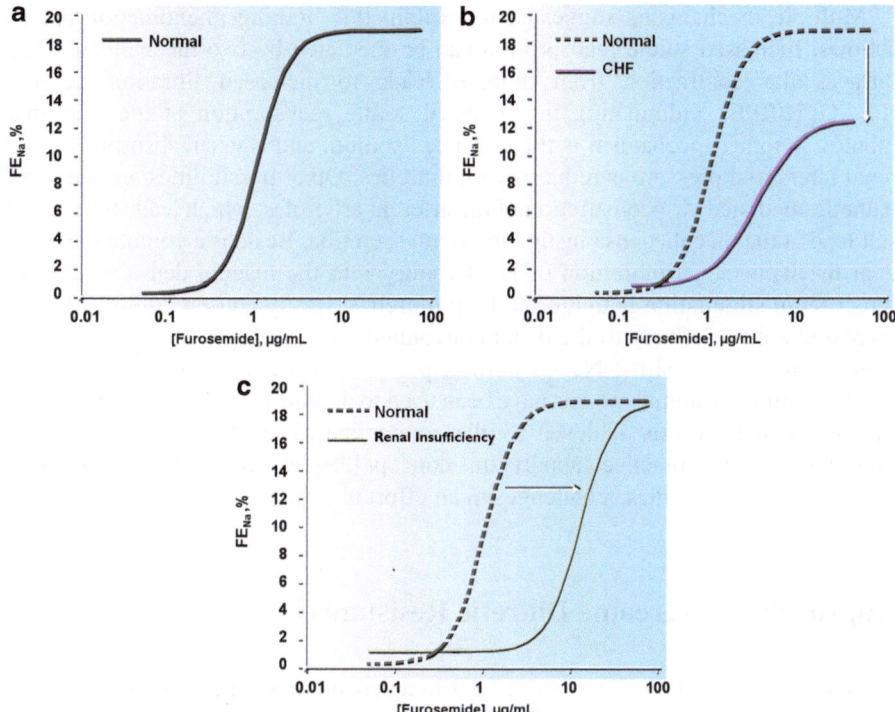

Fig. 3 Pharmacodynamic property of loop diuretic showing the natriuretic response to tubular concentration of the drug. Adapted from Brater [35]

Table 1 Recommended dosing of diuretics in the setting of heart failure with renal insufficiency

Drug (dose in mg)	Heart failure with renal insufficiency		Heart failure with no renal impairment
	Moderate	Severe	
Furosemide	80–160	160–200	40–80
Toresemide	20–50	50–100	10–20
Bumetanide	4–8	8–10	1–2

Once drug levels in the tubular fluid falls below the threshold limit as described earlier, natriuresis is halted and instead a compensatory phase of sodium retention begins until further administration of the drug causes optimal drug levels. This is called post-diuretic sodium chloride retention. Almost all the sodium lost during natriuresis can be reclaimed, especially in the absence of sodium restriction [37]. Hence, it is imperative to emphasize dietary regulation of sodium, if a net negative salt balance is to be achieved. Also of interest is the new steady state noted when loop diuretics are administered on a chronic basis. A chronic adaptation tends to occur as evident by the reduced natriuresis following diuretic dose, commonly described as diuretic braking or diuretic resistance [38].

Multiple mechanisms suggested to explain this braking phenomenon are as follows. Increased solute reabsorption can be mediated by two mechanisms. The intravascular contraction from diuresis leads to increased filtration fraction (FF=GFR/RPF), culminating in enhanced solute reabsorption at the proximal tubules. Another mechanism is the enhanced sodium and water reabsorption once renal interstitial pressure is reduced with diuretics. Other possibilities are the sympathetic-mediated vasoconstriction of the afferent arterioles, which leads to reduced salt load at the macula densa instigating renin secretion. Besides a volume independent mechanism via inhibition of Na–Cl entry into the macula densa leading to direct renin stimulation is unique to loop diuretics. Lastly and predominantly, the increased solute delivery to the distal convoluted tubules causes increased expression of thiazide sensitive Na–Cl co-transporters, which facilitates avid sodium uptake. Although animal models have been used to demonstrate this cellular change, the augmented diuresis achieved by the concomitant use of thiazides with loop diuretics in clinical practice supports this concept [39]. Hence, strategies have been tailored to overcome these challenges in an effort to achieve adequate natriuresis.

Approach to Overcome Diuretic Resistance

An adequate clinical response to diuretics in an edematous state such as congestive HF is a goal of weight loss of at least 1 kg/day. In the absence of salt restriction, diuretic induced natriuresis may not bring about an ECF volume contraction. Hence, the initial focus would be to restrict sodium intake.

Combination Therapy

Drugs such as thiazides and carbonic anhydrous inhibitors have been shown to have a synergistic effect when combined with loop diuretics [40]. The plausible mechanism for this could be one of the following described below. Since most DCT diuretics have a longer half-life compared to loop diuretics, they tend to mitigate the post-diuretic retention of sodium, since they continue to exert a negative sodium balance, even in the absence of loop diuretic in the tubular lumen. DCT diuretics can also hamper sodium reabsorption along the PCT during volume contracted states, via inhibition of the carbonic anhydrase enzyme. Lastly, the ability of DCT diuretics to inhibit the thiazide sensitive Na–Cl co-transporter channels counteracts the adaptive hypertrophy noted in distal nephrons (with chronic loop diuretic use), which otherwise causes up to a threefold increase in sodium chloride reabsorption. Hence, it is appropriate to add a long-acting agent such as metolazone to the existing loop diuretic regimen. Although comparative analyses with shorter acting thiazide agents have not revealed significant benefit of one over the other, the potency of this combination can result in significant electrolyte imbalance and volume contraction that can be a challenge in itself [41]. Given that short duration of combination therapy is as effective as or safer than prolonged courses, most clinicians suggest an initial robust dosing followed by a transition to loop diuretics alone. Alternate approach would be to use other agents such as PCT diuretics or diuretics that act on the collecting duct. Aldosterone antagonists which belong to the latter group have the added advantage that they have been shown to improve mortality, even if they have limited synergistic effect with regard to natriuresis [13, 14].

Continuous Infusion

The major advantage offered by continuous infusion is the avoidance of post-diuretic sodium chloride absorption that occurs during trough levels. However, a greater efficacy was observed with continuous rather than bolus dosing probably due to a smooth, more constant effect relative to drug levels in the urine [42, 43]. As an added advantage, untoward side effects such as ototoxicity and myopathy (in the case of bumetanide) are less likely to occur in the continuous infusion group given that peak levels attained are much lower than in bolus technique.

Although loop diuretics can induce natriuresis, the urine tends to be hypotonic and causes release of adrenergic hormones via stimulation of the RAAS. Of late, there is increased interest in fluid removal via extracorporeal techniques, in an effort to restore the preload condition to the "optimal" zone in the Frank–Starling curve. UF is one such modality which lowered filling pressures and "levels of neurohormones (such as norepinephrine, renin, and aldosterone) with better clinical outcomes". The rationale and evidence of such an approach is discussed below.

Ultrafiltration: Mechanism

The mechanical removal of fluid in congested states has been successfully executed by nephrologists via peritoneal and hemodialysis techniques. UF offers the unique advantage of removing isotonic fluid by generating a convective gradient across a semipermeable membrane. The filtered blood is returned to circulation via a venous access. With an active removal of fluid in this manner, the vascular compartment gets refilled because of the movement of solvent from the extracellular space, enabling a reduction of congestion or edema. The plasma refill rate (PRR) is a compensatory answer to the filtered volume loss and is dependent on the interstitial, serum oncotic and capillary hydrostatic pressure. However, if there is accelerated filtering, the PRR is unable to maintain the equilibrium, causing intravascular volume depletion and stimulation of the neurohormones. The success in the implementation of UF lies in the concept of reducing salt and water load while maintaining an adequate intravascular compartment (Fig. 4).

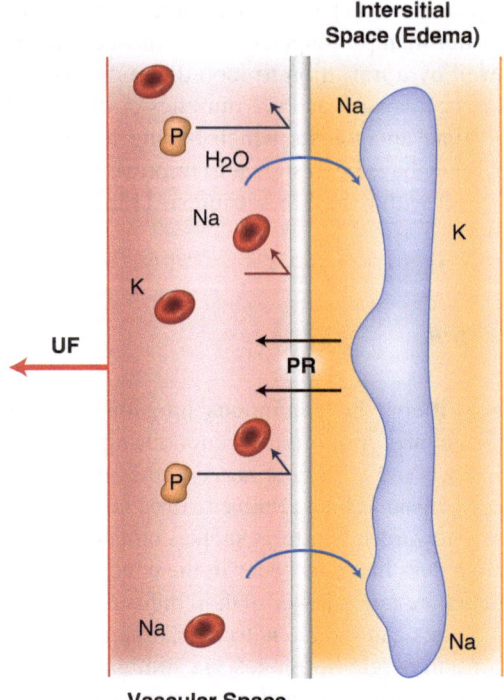

Fig. 4 Basic sketch elaborating the concept of ultrafiltration. Hypervolemia from activation of renin–angiotensin–aldosterone system (RAAS) axis results in movement of water molecules into the interstitial space causing edema (*blue curved arrow*). During ultrafiltration, plasma is forced across a membrane facilitating the movement of water and solutes across the filter guided by a transmembrane pressure gradient. This initiates movement of isotonic fluid from the interstitial space into the vascular compartment. This flow, otherwise called plasma refill (PR), maintains the integrity of the intravascular compartment, at the same time aiding net loss of sodium and water. Courtesy of Gambro UF Solutions, Inc

UF: History and Rationale for Application

Although the concept of mechanical fluid removal was proposed about half a century ago, it was put into application in the 1970s by Silverstein and later by Paganini [44, 45]. When applied to patients with refractory HF, symptomatic relief was correlated with reduction of filling pressures in both right and left chambers of the heart [46]. The weight reduction produced with fluid loss was shown to extend up to a week following discharge [47]. This benefit was attributed to an improvement in diuretic response following UF. The possibility of large volume removal in the range of 500 mL/h offering relief of congestive symptoms without derangement of intravascular volume opened the gates for a renewed interest this approach.

Through the 1990s, the work of Agostini and his group laid the ground work for the modern use of UF in HF therapy. In a randomized controlled trial, they divided

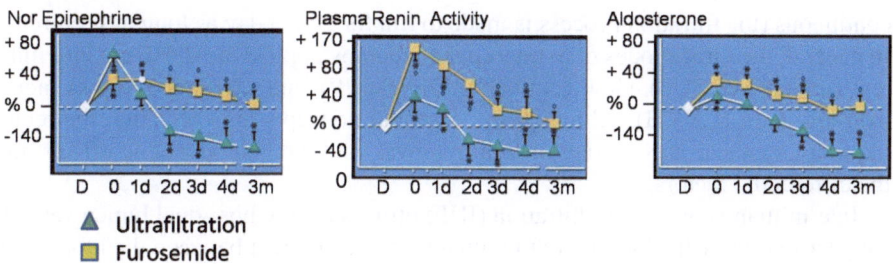

Fig. 5 Correlation of neurohormone levels to UF/diuretic therapy. Data derived from [48]

16 patients with moderate HF on standardized regimen into two groups. The "case" group was subjected to UF and the "control" was given supplemental intravenous doses of furosemide, with the intent to remove an average of 1,600 mL of fluid in both groups. The results revealed that despite a reduction of ventricular filling pressures and body weight, plasma renin activity, norepinephrine, and aldosterone were augmented in the diuretic group. This finding noted in the immediate treatment period persisted for the next 4 days with the patient returning to a fluid congested state (with no improvement in functional capacity). However in the "case" group who received UF, levels of neurohormones fell to below control values within the first 48 h lasting up to 3 months after the initial UF (refer to Fig. 5) [48]. The decrease in fluid intake and diminutive diuretic response in the absence of weight gain suggested the establishment of a new set point in the hypothalamus for water metabolism. Given an equivalent removal of fluid in both the groups, the varying outcome could possibly be due to difference in the solute content of the two fluids. UF leads to an isotonic fluid removal, which suggests an approximate 150 mmol of sodium loss for every 1,000 mL of ultrafiltrate, when compared to 100 mmol under the influence of furosemide [49]. The altered neurohormonal response noted could be owed to a variation of net sodium loss, with an isotonic extraction enabling a more favorable outcome (Fig. 5).

Marenzi et al. utilized UF in 32 patients with NYHA classes II–IV HF who were divided into three groups. They observed that sodium loss and diuresis was inversely related to combination of factors such as neurohormones (such as renin, aldosterone) and renal perfusion pressure. In those with no evidence of overhydration, who maintained relatively good urine output (urine output >1,000 mL/24 h), volume removal caused an increment in the measure of neurohormones. However in the setting of hypervolemia, irrespective of initial urinary output, reduction of neurohormones was noted [50]. It is speculative to conclude that alleviation of hypervolemia resulted in a better neurohormonal level because of the enhanced clearance of norepinephrine through improved diuresis. Blake and their group hypothesized the removal of a cardiac toxin by UF as an explanation for improvement in cardiac function, giving this technique a unique superiority over other measures to relieve congestion [51].

With a wider acceptance of this technology, based on their duration and frequency, UF application was grouped as isolated (single session of 2–4 h), intermittent (single sessions of 2–4 h repeated daily or three times a week for a specific period), and continuous (the filtration process is made to run for 24 h a day as long as required). In general, the three modes of extracorporeal therapy applied in ADHF are intermittent isolated UF (IUF), slow continuous UF (SCUF), and Continuous venovenous hemofiltration (CVVH). Although the essential concepts are the same, the technique for vascular access, rate of fluid removal, and the hemodynamic effects are the differential factors.

Intermittent isolated ultrafiltration (IUF) utilizes a large bore dual lumen venous catheter to establish a blood circuit with a pressure gradient between the blood and UF compartment. The isotonic filtrate removed in sessions every 1–4 h enables large volume removal. Although they appear to be an effective strategy in refractory HF, there is paucity of data with regard to their use. In a pilot study comprising of only 12 patients with end-stage HF refractory to diuretics, Dormans and his group had limited success in showing sustained benefit following IUF with only seven patients showing improvement of NYHA status from IV to III [52]. In a separate study comprising of similar clinical cohort, a French team under Canaud demonstrated that slow daily UF for 4–8 h and SCUF were effective in improving symptoms and restoring cardiac performance while preserving hemodynamics [53]. The limitations of these studies are the absence of a control group where standard therapy was applied and scarcity of data regarding renal function.

UF: Current Applications

UF procedures in general were noted to be cumbersome with the requirement of a central venous access and monitoring in an intensive care unit under the supervision of nurses who have received specialized training. The large volume extracted via extracorporeal devices usually caused hemodynamic instability and hypotension often restricting patients to their bed. The introduction of a portable system called Aquadex System 100 (CHF Solutions, Brooklyn Park, Minnesota) offered the advantage of allowing SCUF to occur via a peripheral or central venous access. The programmable device can be set to extract fluid at the rate up to 500 mL/h at blood flow rates ranging from 10 to 40 mL/min, which gives it a significant advantage over standard venovenous hemodialysis modalities, which requires considerable higher blood flow rate above 400 mL/h. However, the lack of clearance capabilities limits the use of this device in those who are dialysis dependent (Fig. 6).

The advantage in managing fluid shifts led to UF with Aquadex system as a more commonly deployed technique and better studied for therapeutic applications in HF. Early Ultrafiltration in Patients with Decompensated Heart Failure and Observed Resistance to Intervention with Diuretic Agents (EUPHORIA) study was a single-center prospective analysis evaluating the feasibility and safety of UF utilizing the Aquadex system in reducing length of hospitalization. Twenty HF patients who demonstrated diuretic resistance were subjected to UF prior to any IV diuretics or vaso-active drugs. UF showed an improvement in weight, functional status, and B-type natriuretic peptide levels [54]. The effects were persistent even at 30- and 90-day

Fig. 6 Aquadex Flexflow™ (modified version of Aquadex System 100). Courtesy of Gambro UF Solutions, Inc

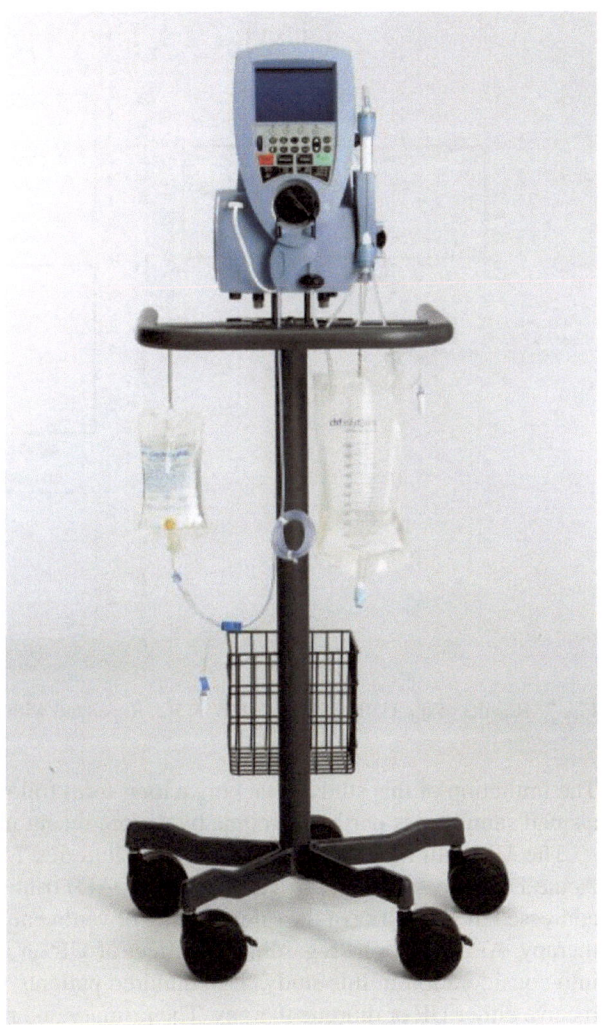

intervals and showed a trend toward decreased hospital stay and rehospitalization. Although there was no comparative analysis that could be performed due to the lack of a control arm, the encouraging reports set the stage for randomized control trials.

The Relief for Acutely Fluid-Overloaded Patients with Decompensated Congestive Heart Failure (RAPID-CHF) Trial was the first randomized controlled trial evaluating the safety and efficacy of UF with the Aquadex system in comparison with standard of care with diuretics at 24 and 48 h, respectively. In this study, Bart et al. showed that the UF group had improved CHF and dyspnea scores with significantly more fluid removal than the diuretic group. Despite patients who underwent UF experiencing more weight loss over the diuretic group (2.5 kg vs. 1.86 kg), the primary end point (24 h weight loss) did not attain a statistical difference [55].

UNLOAD Trial

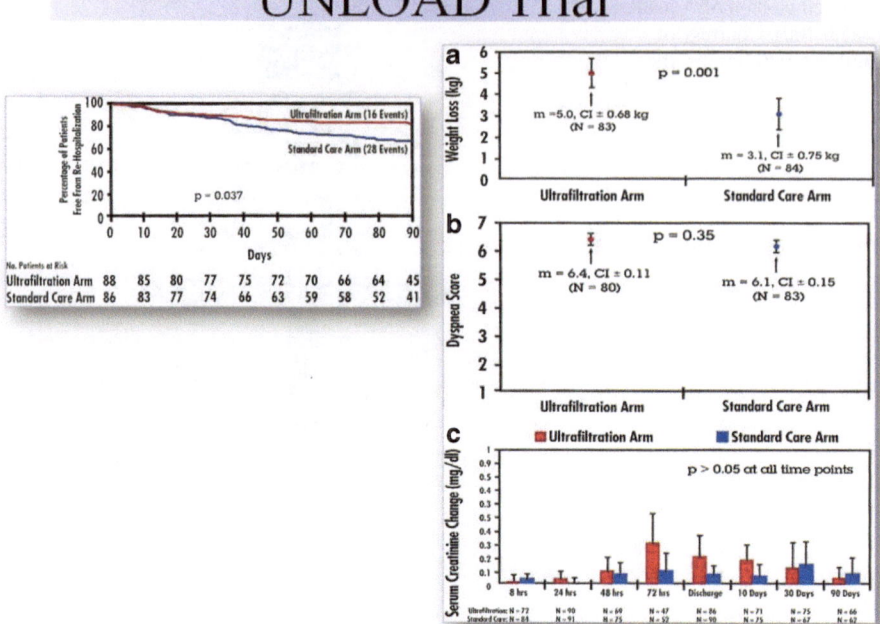

Fig. 7 Results of the UNLOAD trial. From [56]. Reprinted with kind permission from Elsevier

The limitation of this study in lacking a long-term follow-up and being restricted to a small sample was partly overcome by a more recent multicenter trial.

The Ultrafiltration Versus Intravenous Diuretics for Patients Hospitalized for Acute Decompensated Heart Failure (UNLOAD) trial was a landmark trial, which addressed the concerns of the safety profile of venovenous UF over standard diuretic therapy. Also questions regarding the effect of UF on renal parameters were taken into consideration in this study. Two hundred patients were randomized equally to receive either UF or diuretic therapy. The primary end points evaluated at 48 h were weight loss and dyspnea assessment while secondary end points were net fluid loss, rehospitalization for HF, functional capacity, and unscheduled clinic visits in 90 days. The safety profile of the treatment undertaken was measured by evaluating changes in renal parameters, electrolytes, and blood pressure. Patients who received UF had significantly greater weight loss (5 kg vs. 3.1 kg, $p=0.001$) and net fluid loss (4.6 L vs. 3.3 L, $p=0.001$), although the dyspnea scores were similar at 48 h (6.4 vs. 6.1, $p=0.35$). There was less need for rescue therapy with vasoactive agents and as an added benefit, UF allowed patients to take a lower dosage of oral diuretics. A review of these patients at 90 days demonstrated that the effect of fluid loss was evident in decreased need for rehospitalization (18% vs. 32%, $p=0.022$) or visit to physician office or emergency department (21% vs. 44%, $p=0.009$) in the UF group [56]. Thus, the UNLOAD trial clearly showed the benefit of UF as a therapeutic option in ADHF with greater weight and fluid loss in the immediate days following hospitalization and demonstrating continued benefit over 90 days (Fig. 7).

In a separate subanalysis of the diuretic group, there was no statistical difference between the patients who received continuous diuretic infusion and UF when specific target points such as weight loss, net fluid loss and 90-day rehospitalization plus unscheduled physician visits were taken into consideration, although the significance was noted if UF was compared to bolus intravenous diuretics [weight loss: 5 kg vs. 3.6 kg ($p>0.05$) 5 kg vs. 2.9 kg, ($p=0.001$); net fluid loss: 4.6 L vs. 3.9 L ($p>0.05$), 4.6 L vs. 3.1 L ($p<0.001$); rehospitalization equivalent 0.65 vs. 2.29 ($p=0.016$), 0.65 vs. 1.35 ($p=0.05$)].

In a more recent study, Ali et al. evaluated 15 patients with UF who persisted to have congestion despite diuretic treatment. Electrolytes were compared in the ultrafiltrate and the urine sample. There was a significant increase in sodium loss in the ultrafiltrate compared to diuretics (134 ± 8.0 mmol/L vs. 60 ± 47 mmol/L, $p=0.000025$) while net loss of potassium (3.7 ± 0.6 mmol/L vs. 4.1 ± 2.3 mmol/L, $p=0.000017$) and magnesium (2.9 ± 0.7 mg/dL vs. 5.2 ± 3.1 mg/dL, $p=0.017$) was reduced [57]. The question remains as to whether a reduction in total sodium is more favorable over net water deficit in patients who are hypervolemic. Loop diuretics, although effective in reducing congestion, do so by production of hypotonic urine compared to UF, which generates isotonic filtrate. So, there is more "bang for the buck" with UF in regards to total sodium loss. Enabling a net free water deficit in patients with ADHF may improve symptoms in the acute setting but has not offered any mortality benefit as evident from the Efficacy of Vasopressin Antagonism in Heart Failure Trial (EVEREST) [58]. Therefore, it is safe to presume that the long-term benefits associated with HF may be related to neurohormonal activation, which is not worsened while on UF therapy.

In spite of the encouraging findings from the UNLOAD trial, there have been concerns about drawing clinical assumptions. Firstly, neurohormonal profile was not measured in the UNLOAD trial and hence one must be cautious in attributing the lasting benefit observed from UF to the change in neurohormonal levels in the absence of clinical evidence. Secondly, a potential bias is also a concern given the study design that was not blinded. The decision to identify the mode of diuretic administration was left to the physician, whereby those who received continuous loop diuretic infusion were noted to be in higher NYHA class compared to UF, suggesting a cohort that could be sicker, although other cardiovascular parameters (such as left ventricular ejection fraction, BNP levels) were comparable.

Limitations and Future of UF

Firstly, the notable limitation of UF is that in patients who have severe metabolic abnormalities resulting from ADHF and renal dysfunction, SCUF is not a suitable choice, given that there is practically no solute clearance. For these patients, CVVH offers the dual advantage of performing UF and solute removal through a semipermeable membrane via convective transport. This is made possible by filtering a large volume of blood through the chamber but necessitates the use of replacement

Table 2 Comparison of end points from trials using Aquadex Ultrafiltration system

Name of trial	Number of patients	Symptoms	Fluid loss	Weight loss	Change in serum creatinine	Length of stay	Rehospitalization
SAFE	21	–	↓	↓	NS	–	–
EUPHORIA	20	↓	↓	↓	NS	↓	↓
RAPID-CHF	40	↓	NS	↓	NS	NS	–
UNLOAD	200	NS	↓	↓	NS	NS	↓

NS no statistical significance noted. (–) Data not reported in trial

fluid to avoid hemodynamic instability caused by massive fluid shifts. In addition, hemofiltration has been known to remove medium-sized protein, which include certain myocardial toxins such as interkuekin-8 (IL-8) and monocyte chemoattractant protein-1, offering improvement in ejection fraction with reduced diuretic dosing following treatment [59]. In this small study of ten patients, CVVH offered benefit over SCUF; however, there is a need for duplication of benefits through large trials before such a technique can be accepted as a standard of care.

Secondly, the question remains as to what is the ideal fluid removal rate and what is considered an optimal end point once UF is initiated. Previous studies which evaluated the effectiveness of UF utilized time-based approach or symptomatic improvement as their end points. Lucas et al. demonstrated that for ADHF patients in NYHA class IV, improvement in congestive symptoms was associated with improved mortality [60]. Yet, experience with the Aquadex system has not shown consistent results.

As noted in Table 2, UF generates symptomatic relief of statistical significance in the RAPID-CHF trial while this was not the case in the UNLOAD trial, but with regard to weight loss, RAPID-CHF trial produced significant result in comparison to the UNLOAD cohort. Similarly, UNLOAD and EUPHORIA data supported the notion that UF could reduce hospital readmission rates but with regard to length of stay, only EUPHORIA trial revealed any evidence of statistical significance. The lack of a universal approach to fluid removal (single episode of high volume removal as in RAPID-CHF trial, slow continuous UF in UNLOAD) could explain the variation noted in these trials using the same device.

Since clinical signs alone are unreliable indicators of congestive states, attempt to identify euvolemia is pivotal to avoid adverse effects from excessive fluid depletion from intravascular compartment [61]. In an effort to answer this question, Treatment to Euvolemia by Assessment and Measured Blood Volume in Heart Failure (TEAM-HF) trial is currently evaluating the use of blood volume measurements to guide UF in order to improve outcomes.

Another impasse a clinician faces is whether UF can be safely utilized in patients who present with poor renal function but not yet dependent on hemodialysis. Analyzing the data from the various trials, patients who were enrolled to the trials had a mean creatinine less than 2.5 mg/dL and those who received UF showed minimal increase in serum creatinine, although the change was not rendered significant enough to be considered as an adverse outcome (refer to Fig. 8). Hence,

Creatinine variation from baseline following Ultrafiltration

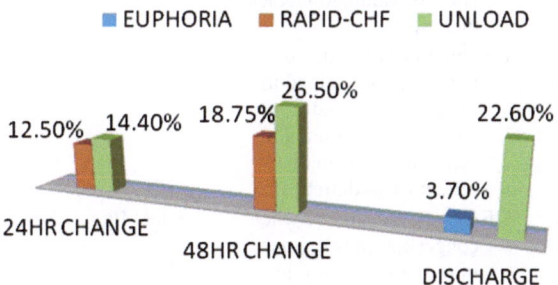

Fig. 8 Percentage change in serum creatinine from baseline following ultrafiltration in recent trials

the challenge of advocating UF in patients who manifest in cardiorenal syndrome needs further scrutiny. A National Heart, Lung and Blood Institute (NHLBI) sponsored study (Cardiorenal Rescue Study in Acute Decompensated Heart Failure: CARRESS) is underway to evaluate this high risk group, although patients with serum creatinine greater than 3.5 mg/dL are excluded from this trial.

Lastly, the dispute over the cost-effectiveness of this approach is relevant, especially in an era where the major changes are advocated in an effort to curb expenses related to patient care. HF treatment is the single costliest (15% of total cost) diagnosis related group (DRG) on Medicare claims [62]. In an effort to analyze the cost-effectiveness of UF compared to diuretics, Bradley and their group applied a decision-analytic model to patients enrolled in the UNLOAD trial. From a societal perspective, the total cost incurred in UF at index hospitalization and follow-up at 90 days added up to $13,469 when compared to $11,610 in the diuretic group [63]. Rehospitalization contributed to a 39% of the total cost in those who received diuretics while it only contributed to 18% in the UF arm. Given that rehospitalization was notably lower in the UF arm, it was cost-saving in 99% of iterations from a Medicare perspective but given the use of a DRG-based reimbursements, additional costs encountered with use of UF therapy are not recovered from a hospital point of view. The study concluded that UF was unlikely to be a cost-effective choice over diuretics from a societal point of consideration. Recently, Ross and Kazory suggested a variation to the above in order to reduce cost. In their opinion, if conventional devices and filters are to be utilized, the likelihood of this approach to be financially viable was more certain. When the same cost analysis design was applied in their proposed model, the total costs tilted in favor of UF ($11,293 for UF vs. $11,610 for diuretics), thus advocating the possibility that modifications in the extracorporeal circuit can be a place for future research [64].

In summary, the syndrome of ADHF with coexistent renal dysfunction is a common presentation which in summation increases mortality. The application of diuretics may be significantly limited by diuretic resistance or adverse effects related

Table 3 Current guidelines for the use of ultrafiltration for ADHF

AHA/ACC practice guideline (2009)	UF is reasonable for patients with refractory congestion, not responding to medical therapy	Class IIa	Level of evidence: B
European Society of Cardiology (2008)	UF should be considered to reduce fluid overload in select patients and to correct hyponatremia in symptomatic patients, refractory to diuretics	Class IIa	Level of evidence: B
Heart Failure Society of America (2010)	UF may be considered when congestion fails to improve in response to diuretics	Class IIa	Level of evidence: C

to their use. With the advent of mechanical removal of isotonic fluid via peripherally inserted catheters through SCUF modalities, patients have been observed to have reduced rehospitalization and sustained clinical benefit. Current use of UF is restricted to a limited group of patients with ADHF who are not responding to medical therapy (refer to Table 3). Physicians will need to carefully identify the ideal cohort of patients and evaluate the risk benefit ratio of this approach, while considering the cost-effectiveness over conventional approach. With more acceptance of this application and data from ongoing trials, some of these concerns can be addressed and enable the physician to use a potentially new tool.

References

1. Writing Group Members, Lloyd-Jones D, Adams RJ, et al. Heart disease and stroke statistics—2010 update: a report from the American Heart Association. Circulation. 2010;121(7):e46–215.
2. Adams Jr KF, Fonarow GC, Emerman CL, et al. Characteristics and outcomes of patients hospitalized for heart failure in the United States: rationale, design, and preliminary observations from the first 100,000 cases in the Acute Decompensated Heart Failure National Registry (ADHERE). Am Heart J. 2005;149(2):209–16.
3. O'Connor CM, Stough WG, Gallup DS, Hasselblad V, Gheorghiade M. Demographics, clinical characteristics, and outcomes of patients hospitalized for decompensated heart failure: observations from the IMPACT-HF registry. J Card Fail. 2005;11(3):200–5.
4. Metra M, Nodari S, Parrinello G, et al. Worsening renal function in patients hospitalised for acute heart failure: clinical implications and prognostic significance. Eur J Heart Fail. 2008;10(2):188–95.
5. Cleland JG, Swedberg K, Follath F, et al. The EuroHeart Failure survey programme—a survey on the quality of care among patients with heart failure in Europe. Part 1: patient characteristics and diagnosis. Eur Heart J. 2003;24(5):442–63.
6. Fonarow GC, Abraham WT, Albert NM, et al. Organized Program to Initiate Lifesaving Treatment in Hospitalized Patients with Heart Failure (OPTIMIZE-HF): rationale and design. Am Heart J. 2004;148(1):43–51.
7. Nieminen MS, Bohm M, Cowie MR, et al. Executive summary of the guidelines on the diagnosis and treatment of acute heart failure: the Task Force on Acute Heart Failure of the European Society of Cardiology. Eur Heart J. 2005;26(4):384–416.

8. Krumholz HM, Keenan PS, Brush Jr JE, et al. Standards for measures used for public reporting of efficiency in health care: a scientific statement from the American Heart Association Interdisciplinary Council on Quality of Care and Outcomes Research and the American College of Cardiology Foundation. Circulation. 2008;118(18):1885–93.
9. Schrier RW, Berl T. Nonosmolar factors affecting renal water excretion (first of two parts). N Engl J Med. 1975;292(2):81–8.
10. Schrier RW, Cadnapaphornchai MA, Umenishi F. Water-losing and water-retaining states: role of water channels and vasopressin receptor antagonists. Heart Dis. 2001;3(3):210–4.
11. De Angelis N, Fiordaliso F, Latini R, et al. Appraisal of the role of angiotensin II and aldosterone in ventricular myocyte apoptosis in adult normotensive rat. J Mol Cell Cardiol. 2002;34(12):1655–65.
12. Rocha R, Stier Jr CT, Kifor I, et al. Aldosterone: a mediator of myocardial necrosis and renal arteriopathy. Endocrinology. 2000;141(10):3871–8.
13. Pitt B, Zannad F, Remme WJ, et al. The effect of spironolactone on morbidity and mortality in patients with severe heart failure. Randomized Aldactone Evaluation Study Investigators. N Engl J Med. 1999;341(10):709–17.
14. Pitt B, Remme W, Zannad F, et al. Eplerenone, a selective aldosterone blocker, in patients with left ventricular dysfunction after myocardial infarction. N Engl J Med. 2003;348(14):1309–21.
15. Forman DE, Butler J, Wang Y, et al. Incidence, predictors at admission, and impact of worsening renal function among patients hospitalized with heart failure. J Am Coll Cardiol. 2004;43(1): 61–7.
16. Damman K, Navis G, Voors AA, et al. Worsening renal function and prognosis in heart failure: systematic review and meta-analysis. J Card Fail. 2007;13(8):599–608.
17. Ljungman S, Laragh JH, Cody RJ. Role of the kidney in congestive heart failure. Relationship of cardiac index to kidney function. Drugs. 1990;39 Suppl 4:10–21 [discussion 22–4].
18. Maxwell MH, Breed ES, Schwartz IL. Renal venous pressure in chronic congestive heart failure. J Clin Invest. 1950;29(3):342–8.
19. Kastner PR, Hall JE, Guyton AC. Renal hemodynamic responses to increased renal venous pressure: role of angiotensin II. Am J Physiol. 1982;243(3):F260–4.
20. Charloux A, Piquard F, Doutreleau S, Brandenberger G, Geny B. Mechanisms of renal hyporesponsiveness to ANP in heart failure. Eur J Clin Invest. 2003;33(9):769–78.
21. Morsing P, Stenberg A, Casellas D, et al. Renal interstitial pressure and tubuloglomerular feedback control in rats during infusion of atrial natriuretic peptide (ANP). Acta Physiol Scand. 1992;146(3):393–8.
22. Firth JD, Raine AEG, Ledingham JGG. Raised venous pressure: a direct cause of renal sodium retention in oedema? Lancet. 1988;331(8593):1033–6.
23. Morley D, Brozena SC. Assessing risk by hemodynamic profile in patients awaiting cardiac transplantation. Am J Cardiol. 1994;73(5):379–83.
24. Unverferth DV, Magorien RD, Moeschberger ML, Baker PB, Fetters JK, Leier CV. Factors influencing the one-year mortality of dilated cardiomyopathy. Am J Cardiol. 1984; 54(1):147–52.
25. Damman K, Navis G, Smilde TD, et al. Decreased cardiac output, venous congestion and the association with renal impairment in patients with cardiac dysfunction. Eur J Heart Fail. 2007;9(9):872–8.
26. Damman K, van Deursen VM, Navis G, Voors AA, van Veldhuisen DJ, Hillege HL. Increased central venous pressure is associated with impaired renal function and mortality in a broad spectrum of patients with cardiovascular disease. J Am Coll Cardiol. 2009;53(7):582–8.
27. Binanay C, Califf RM, Hasselblad V, et al. Evaluation study of congestive heart failure and pulmonary artery catheterization effectiveness: the ESCAPE trial. JAMA. 2005;294(13):1625–33.
28. Nohria A, Hasselblad V, Stebbins A, et al. Cardiorenal interactions: insights from the ESCAPE trial. J Am Coll Cardiol. 2008;51(13):1268–74.
29. Mullens W, Abrahams Z, Francis GS, et al. Importance of venous congestion for worsening of renal function in advanced decompensated heart failure. J Am Coll Cardiol. 2009;53(7): 589–96.

30. Patterson JH, Adams Jr KF, Applefeld MM, Corder CN, Masse BR. Oral torsemide in patients with chronic congestive heart failure: effects on body weight, edema, and electrolyte excretion. Torsemide Investigators Group. Pharmacotherapy. 1994;14(5):514–21.
31. Sherman LG, Liang CS, Baumgardner S, Charuzi Y, Chardo F, Kim CS. Piretanide, a potent diuretic with potassium-sparing properties, for the treatment of congestive heart failure. Clin Pharmacol Ther. 1986;40(5):587–94.
32. Kramer BK, Schweda F, Riegger GA. Diuretic treatment and diuretic resistance in heart failure. Am J Med. 1999;106(1):90–6.
33. Faris Rajaa F, Flather M, Purcell H, Poole-Wilson PA, Coats Andrew JS. Diuretics for heart failure. Cochrane Database Syst Rev. 2006;(1). http://www.mrw.interscience.wiley.com/cochrane/clsysrev/articles/CD003838/frame.html.
34. McCurley JM, Hanlon SU, Wei SK, Wedam EF, Michalski M, Haigney MC. Furosemide and the progression of left ventricular dysfunction in experimental heart failure. J Am Coll Cardiol. 2004;44(6):1301–7.
35. Brater DC. Diuretic therapy. N Engl J Med. 1998;339(6):387–95.
36. Vargish T, Benjamin R, Shenkman L. Deafness from furosemide. Ann Intern Med. 1970; 72(5):761.
37. Ellison DH. Diuretic therapy and resistance in congestive heart failure. Cardiology. 2001; 96(3–4):132–43.
38. Wilcox CS, Mitch WE, Kelly RA, et al. Response of the kidney to furosemide. I. Effects of salt intake and renal compensation. J Lab Clin Med. 1983;102(3):450–8.
39. Knauf H, Mutschler E. Functional state of the nephron and diuretic dose-response—rationale for low-dose combination therapy. Cardiology. 1994;84 Suppl 2:18–26.
40. Ellison DH. The physiologic basis of diuretic synergism: its role in treating diuretic resistance. Ann Intern Med. 1991;114(10):886–94.
41. Channer KS, McLean KA, Lawson-Matthew P, Richardson M. Combination diuretic treatment in severe heart failure: a randomised controlled trial. Br Heart J. 1994;71(2):146–50.
42. Dormans TP, van Meyel JJ, Gerlag PG, Tan Y, Russel FG, Smits P. Diuretic efficacy of high dose furosemide in severe heart failure: bolus injection versus continuous infusion. J Am Coll Cardiol. 1996;28(2):376–82.
43. Kramer WG, Smith WB, Ferguson J, et al. Pharmacodynamics of torsemide administered as an intravenous injection and as a continuous infusion to patients with congestive heart failure. J Clin Pharmacol. 1996;36(3):265–70.
44. Silverstein ME, Ford CA, Lysaght MJ, Henderson LW. Treatment of severe fluid overload by ultrafiltration. N Engl J Med. 1974;291(15):747–51.
45. Paganini EP, Fouad F, Tarazi RC, Bravo EL, Nakamoto S. Hemodynamics of isolated ultrafiltration in chronic hemodialysis patients. Trans Am Soc Artif Intern Organs. 1979;25: 422–5.
46. Rimondini A, Cipolla CM, Della Bella P, et al. Hemofiltration as short-term treatment for refractory congestive heart failure. Am J Med. 1987;83(1):43–8.
47. Simpson IA, Simpson K, Rae AP, Boulton-Jones JM, Allison ME, Hutton I. Ultrafiltration in diuretic-resistant cardiac failure. Ren Fail. 1987;10(2):115–9.
48. Agostoni P, Marenzi G, Lauri G, et al. Sustained improvement in functional capacity after removal of body fluid with isolated ultrafiltration in chronic cardiac insufficiency: failure of furosemide to provide the same result. Am J Med. 1994;96(3):191–9.
49. Canaud B, Leray-Moragues H, Garred LJ, et al. Slow isolated ultrafiltration for the treatment of congestive heart failure. Am J Kidney Dis. 1996;28(5):S67–73.
50. Marenzi G, Grazi S, Giraldi F, et al. Interrelation of humoral factors, hemodynamics, and fluid and salt metabolism in congestive heart failure: effects of extracorporeal ultrafiltration. Am J Med. 1993;94(1):49–56.
51. Blake P, Hasegawa Y, Khosla MC, Fouad-Tarazi F, Sakura N, Paganini EP. Isolation of "myocardial depressant factor(s)" from the ultrafiltrate of heart failure patients with acute renal failure. ASAIO J. 1996;42(5):M911–5.

52. Dormans TP, Huige RM, Gerlag PG. Chronic intermittent haemofiltration and haemodialysis in end stage chronic heart failure with oedema refractory to high dose frusemide. Heart. 1996;75(4):349–51.
53. Canaud B, Leblanc M, Leray-Moragues H, Delmas S, Klouche K, Beraud JJ. Slow continuous and daily ultrafiltration for refractory congestive heart failure. Nephrol Dial Transplant. 1998;13 Suppl 4:51–5.
54. Costanzo MR, Saltzberg M, O'Sullivan J, Sobotka P. Early ultrafiltration in patients with decompensated heart failure and diuretic resistance. J Am Coll Cardiol. 2005;46(11):2047–51.
55. Bart BA, Boyle A, Bank AJ, et al. Ultrafiltration versus usual care for hospitalized patients with heart failure: the Relief for Acutely Fluid-Overloaded Patients With Decompensated Congestive Heart Failure (RAPID-CHF) trial. J Am Coll Cardiol. 2005;46(11):2043–6.
56. Costanzo MR, Guglin ME, Saltzberg MT, et al. Ultrafiltration versus intravenous diuretics for patients hospitalized for acute decompensated heart failure. J Am Coll Cardiol. 2007; 49(6):675–83.
57. Ali SS, Olinger CC, Sobotka PA, et al. Loop diuretics can cause clinical natriuretic failure: a prescription for volume expansion. Congest Heart Fail. 2009;15(1):1–4.
58. Konstam MA, Gheorghiade M, Burnett Jr JC, et al. Effects of oral tolvaptan in patients hospitalized for worsening heart failure: the EVEREST Outcome Trial. JAMA. 2007;297(12):1319–31.
59. Libetta C, Sepe V, Zucchi M, et al. Intermittent haemodiafiltration in refractory congestive heart failure: BNP and balance of inflammatory cytokines. Nephrol Dial Transplant. 2007;22(7):2013–9.
60. Lucas C, Johnson W, Hamilton MA, et al. Freedom from congestion predicts good survival despite previous class IV symptoms of heart failure. Am Heart J. 2000;140(6):840–7.
61. Chakko S, Woska D, Martinez H, et al. Clinical, radiographic, and hemodynamic correlations in chronic congestive heart failure: conflicting results may lead to inappropriate care. Am J Med. 1991;90(3):353–9.
62. Whellan DJ, Greiner MA, Schulman KA, Curtis LH. Costs of inpatient care among Medicare beneficiaries with heart failure, 2001 to 2004. Circ Cardiovasc Qual Outcomes. 2010;3(1): 33–40.
63. Bradley SM, Levy WC, Veenstra DL. Cost-consequences of ultrafiltration for acute heart failure: a decision model analysis. Circ Cardiovasc Qual Outcomes. 2009;2(6):566–73.
64. Ross EA, Kazory A. Overcoming financial constraints of ultrafiltration for heart failure. Am J Cardiol. 2010;105(10):1504–5.

Index

A

ACE. *See* Angiotensin-converting enzyme (ACE)

Acute decompensated heart failure (ADHF)
  acute coronary syndrome, 91
  ADHERE, 96
  cardiovascular disease management, 91
  clinical syndrome, 91
  congestion, 86
  IUF, 102
  pathophysiology, hypervolemia, 92–94
  RAAS, 92
  renal function, 94
  renal venous pressure, 76
  UNLOAD trial, 104

Acute Decompensated Heart Failure National Registry (ADHERE), 1, 4, 5, 24, 92, 96

ADHERE. *See* Acute Decompensated Heart Failure National Registry (ADHERE)

ADHF. *See* Acute decompensated heart failure (ADHF)

AHA. *See* American Heart Association (AHA)

Aldosterone antagonists
  ACC/AHA indications, 15
  EPHESUS, 14
  RALES, 14–15
  RAS inhibitors, 16
  sodium excretion, 14

Aldosterone receptor antagonists (ARAs)
  EPHESUS, 35
  hyperkalemia, 35
  spironolactone and eplerenone, 34

Aliskiren Observation of Heart Failure Treatment (ALOFT) study, 36

ALLHAT. *See* Anti-hypertensive and lipid-lowering treatment to prevent heart attack trial (ALLHAT)

ALOFT study. *See* Aliskiren Observation of Heart Failure Treatment (ALOFT) study

American Heart Association (AHA), 15, 17

Analysis of the National Health and Nutritional Examination Survey (NHANES), 59

Angiotensin-converting enzyme (ACE) inhibitors, 6, 12, 13
  CONSENSUS trial, 27
  hyperkalemia, 29
  SOLVD trials, 28

Angiotensin receptor blockers (ARBs), 6
  ACE inhibitor, 32
  and angiotensin-converting enzyme inhibitor, 66–67
  CHARM, 29–30
  CKD, 32
  and direct renin inhibitor, 65
  ELITE, 13
  hyperkalemia, 31–32
  inhibitors, 12, 13
  OPTIMAAL, 29
  proteinuria, 14
  RESOLVD, 13
  serum potassium, 33
  spironolactone, 30
  Val-HeFT, 13, 29

Anglo-scandinavian cardiac outcomes trial (ASCOT), 64

Anti-hypertensive and lipid-lowering treatment to prevent heart attack trial (ALLHAT), 60

G.L. Bakris (ed.), *Managing the Kidney when the Heart is Failing*,
DOI 10.1007/978-1-4614-3691-1, © Springer Science+Business Media New York 2012

ARAs. *See* Aldosterone receptor antagonists
    (ARAs)
ARBs. *See* Angiotensin receptor
    blockers (ARBs)
Arginine vasopressin (AVP), 92, 93
ASCOT. *See* Anglo-Scandinavian cardiac
    outcomes trial (ASCOT)
Atherosclerosis
    disordered bone and mineral
        metabolism, 46
    RAS, 44, 54
AVP. *See* Arginine vasopressin (AVP)

B
Blood pressure (BP), 59
BP. *See* Blood pressure (BP)

C
Calcium channel blockers (CCB)
    and beta blocker, 66
    dihydropyridine and
        nondihydropyridine, 66
    and diuretic, 65
    renin–angiotensin–aldosterone inhibitor
        ASCOT, 64
        INVEST, 64
        systolic blood pressure, 64–65
Candesartan in Heart Failure-Assessment
        of Reduction in Mortality
        and Morbidity (CHARM), 29–32
Cardiorenal syndrome, 106–107
Cardiovascular effects of renal artery stenosis
    angiotensin II, 47–48
    diastolic dysfunction, 48
    revascularization reports, 48–51
Centers for Medicare and Medicaid
        Services (CMS), 17
Central venous pressure (CVP), 94
CHARM. *See* Candesartan in Heart
        Failure-Assessment of Reduction in
        Mortality and Morbidity (CHARM)
CHF. *See* Congestive heart failure (CHF)
Chronic kidney disease (CKD), 25, 26, 32
    ADHERE, 5
    atherosclerotic RAS, 45
    cross-sectional studies, 3, 5
    diagnosis
        chronicity, 2
        creatinine, 2
        glomerular filtration, 2, 3
        proteinuria, 3

    renal damage, 2
    stages, 2
    epidemiology, 1–2
    evaluation, 54
    HF patients, 3, 4
    population, 48
    renovascular, 43, 46
    systolic HF, 5, 6
    therapeutic implications
        ACE inhibitors, 6
        ARBs, 6
CKD. *See* Chronic kidney disease (CKD)
Clinical trials for treatment of renovascular
        disease, 57
CMS. *See* Centers for Medicare and Medicaid
        Services (CMS)
Congestive heart failure (CHF), 14
CONSENSUS trial. *See* Cooperative North
        Scandinavian Enalapril Survival
        Study (CONSENSUS) trial
Continuous venovenous hemofiltration
        (CVVH)
    convective transport, 105
    SCUF, 106
Cooperative North Scandinavian
        Enalapril Survival Study
        (CONSENSUS) trial, 27
Creatinine
    HF patients, 17
    RAS blockade, 20, 21
    serum, 19, 20
    systolic blood pressure, 20
CTA. *See* CT angiography (CTA)
CT angiography (CTA), 52
CVP. *See* Central venous pressure (CVP)
CVVH. *See* Continuous venovenous
        hemofiltration (CVVH)

D
Diagnosis related group (DRG), 107
Direct renin inhibitors (DRIs)
    ACE inhibitor, 35
    ALOFT, 36
    biochemical abnormalities, 36
    hypotension and hyperkalemia, 37
    RAAS, 35
Distal protection devices, 57
Diuretic resistance
    combination therapy
        carbonic anhydrase enzyme, 98
        drugs, 98
        natriuresis, 99

congestive HF, 98
continuous infusion, 99
Diuretics, 38
DRG. *See* Diagnosis related group (DRG)
DRIs. *See* Direct renin inhibitors (DRIs)

E
Edema mechanisms, HF
  development
    neurohumoral events, 74
    RAAS, 74–75
    renal function, 74
    SNS, 75–76
  diuretics
    adaptation, 81–82
    carbonic anhydrase inhibitors, 77
    dietitian, 83
    furosemide doses, 84
    loop, 78–79, 84
    meta-analysis, 84
    neurohumoral response, 82–83
    osmotic, 76–77
    pharmacokinetics and
      pharmacodynamics, 83
    potassium-sparing, 79–80
    properties, 85
    refractoriness, 80–81
    resistance, 86
    spironolactone, 85
    thiazide, 77–78
  mechanistic-based treatments, 76
  sodium and water retention, 73
Electrolyte disturbances, 86
ELITE. *See* Evaluation of Losartan
    in the Elderly (ELITE)
EPHESUS. *See* Eplerenone Post-Acute
    Myocardial Infarction Heart
    Failure Efficacy and Survival Study
    (EPHESUS)
Epidemiology
  CKD, 1–2
  HF, 1
  prevalence, 3, 4
Eplerenone Post-Acute Myocardial Infarction
    Heart Failure Efficacy and Survival
    Study (EPHESUS), 14, 15, 35
Evaluation of Losartan in the
    Elderly (ELITE), 13

F
Fixed dose combination
  amiloride, 65
  amlodipine and valsartan, 64

Furosemide
  doses, 84
  infusion, 84
  loop diuretic, 78, 85

G
GFR. *See* Glomerular filtration rate (GFR)
Glomerular filtration rate (GFR), 24, 25, 27,
    74, 80, 94

H
HCTZ. *See* Hydrochlorothiazide (HCTZ)
Heart failure (HF). *See also* Edema
    mechanisms, HF
  CKD (*see* Chronic kidney disease (CKD))
  epidemiology, 1, 44
  intervention
    distal protection devices, 57
    HF, revascularization, 56
    procedural complications, 56
  medical therapy, 54
  pathophysiology, 46–47
  percutaneous intervention, 55
  RAAS blockade, 57
  RAS, 43–48, 52–54
  renovascular disease, 44
  stenting, benefit, 55
  surgical management, 54
  treatment (*see* Hyperkalemia risk and
    treatment, HF)
HF. *See* Heart failure (HF)
Hydrochlorothiazide (HCTZ), 77–78
Hyperkalemia, 20–21
Hyperkalemia risk and treatment, HF
  ACE inhibitors, 27–29
  ARAs, 34–35
  ARBs, 29–33
  description, 23
  dietary interventions, 37
  diuretics, 38
  DRIs, 35–37
  pathophysiology
    ACE inhibitors, 26
    controlling processes, 25
    pharmacotherapy, 26
    potassium excretion, 25–26
    systolic dysfunction, 27
  RAAS inhibitors, 37–38
  renal dysfunction, 24–25
  renin–angiotensin–aldosterone system, 33
  serum potassium and renal function, 37
  VALIANT, 33
  worsening renal function, 34

Hypertension
  adherence, 61
  ALLHAT, 60
  BP, 59
  clinical application, 68
  cost, 61
  efficacy, 61
  LIFE, 60
  NHANES, 59
  polypill, 67–68
  RAAS, 60
  SPC
    classes, 62–66
    effective, 66–67
  STRATHE, 60
  three-drug combination pill, 67
  tolerability, 61
Hypervolemia
  pathophysiology
    AVP, 92, 93
    cardiac filling pressures, 92
    myocardial apoptosis, 93–94
    RAAS, 92
  reduction, neurohormones, 101

I
International Verapamil SR-Trandolapril
    (INVEST), 64
INVEST. See International Verapamil
    SR-Trandolapril (INVEST)

J
JCAHO. See Joint Commission on
    Accreditation of Health Care
    Organizations (JCAHO)
Joint Commission on Accreditation of Health
    Care Organizations (JCAHO), 17

L
LIFE. See Losartan intervention
    for endpoints trial (LIFE)
Loop diuretics
  ADHERE, 96
  "braking phenomenon", 79
  furosemide, 79
  HF, renal insufficiency, 96, 97
  PCT, 96
  pharmacodynamic property, 96, 97
  renin secretion, 98
  solute reabsorption, 98
  therapeutic effect, 96

  tubular fluid, 97
  tubular secretion, 78–79
  urinary sodium excretion, 95
Losartan intervention for endpoints trial
    (LIFE), 60

M
Magnetic resonance angiography (MRA), 52
Metolazone
  defined, 78
  loop diuretic, 85
MRA. See Magnetic resonance
    angiography (MRA)

N
NHANES. See Analysis of the National Health
    and Nutritional Examination Survey
    (NHANES)
Nonsteroidal antiinflammatory drugs
    (NSAIDs), 94
NSAIDs. See Nonsteroidal antiinflammatory
    drugs (NSAIDs)

O
OPTIMAAL. See Optimal Trial in Myocardial
    Infarction with the Angiotensin II
    Antagonist Losartan (OPTIMAAL)
Optimal Trial in Myocardial Infarction with
    the Angiotensin II Antagonist
    Losartan (OPTIMAAL), 29

P
PCT. See Proximal convoluted tubule (PCT)
PCWP. See Pulmonary capillary wedge
    pressure (PCWP)
Plasma refill rate (PRR), 99
Proteinuria, 14
Proximal convoluted tubule (PCT), 96
PRR. See Plasma refill rate (PRR)
Pulmonary capillary wedge pressure (PCWP)
  clinical congestion, 92
  venodilatory property, 95

R
RAAS. See Renin-angiotensin-aldosterone
    system (RAAS)
RALES. See Randomized Aldactone
    Evaluation Study Investigators
    (RALES)

Randomized Aldactone Evaluation Study
        Investigators (RALES), 14–15
Randomized evaluation of strategies for left
        ventricular dysfunction
        (RESOLVD), 13
RAP. *See* Right atrial pressure (RAP)
RAS. *See* Renal artery stenosis (RAS)
RAS blockade. *See* Renin–angiotensin system
        (RAS) blockade
RBF. *See* Renal blood flow (RBF)
Renal artery imaging, 52
Renal artery stenosis (RAS)
        defined, 43–44
        imaging, diagnosis, 48, 52–53
        outcomes, atherosclerotic
                cardiovascular events, 45
                HF, 45
                incidental (asymptomatic), 46
        presentation, 48, 52
        renal function, 47
        revascularization *vs.* medical therapy,
                53–54
Renal artery stenting
        defined, 55
        outcomes, kidney function, 55
        "unprotected", 57
Renal blood flow (RBF), 78
Renal dysfunction
        ADHERE, 24
        CKD, 25
        GFR, 24
        proteinuria, 25, 26
Renin-angiotensin-aldosterone system
        (RAAS)
        activation and up-regulation, 46
        administration, 75
        antagonists, 54
        blockade, 54, 57
        inhibitors
                ACE inhibitors, 38
                hyperkalemia, 37
                spironolactone/eplerenone, 38
        kidney, 74
Renin–angiotensin system (RAS) blockade
        ACE inhibitors, 12, 13
        aldosterone antagonists, 14–16
        ARBs, 12–14
        benefits, 17
        clinical syndrome
                complex syndrome, 11
                stages, HF, 12
        hemodynamics
                mechanisms, 17, 19
                neurohumoral systems, 17, 18

        hyperkalemia, 20–21
        renal function worsening
                beta-blocker therapy, 19
                neurohormones, 19
                serum creatinine, 20, 21
                systolic function, 19–20
RESOLVD. *See* Randomized evaluation
        of strategies for left ventricular
        dysfunction (RESOLVD)
Right atrial pressure (RAP), 94

S
Serum potassium and renal function, 37
Single pill combinations (SPCs)
        angiotensin-converting enzyme
                inhibitor and ARB, 66–67
        beta blocker, 67
        classes
                beta blocker and diuretic, 66
                CCB, 65, 66
                direct renin inhibitor and ARB, 65
                drug combinations, hypertension
                        treatment, 62–63
                renin–angiotensin–aldosterone
                        inhibitor, 63–65
                thiazide and potassium-sparing
                        diuretics, 65
        clinical application, 68
        renin–angiotensin–aldosterone inhibitor, 67
SNS. *See* Sympathetic nervous system (SNS)
SOLVD trials. *See* Studies of Left Ventricular
        Dysfunction (SOLVD) trials
Spironolactone, 14, 15, 18
Strategies in treatment of hypertension study
        (STRATHE), 60
STRATHE. *See* Strategies in treatment of
        hypertension study (STRATHE)
Studies of Left Ventricular Dysfunction
        (SOLVD) trials, 28
Sympathetic nervous system (SNS)
        development, HF, 75
        renal venous pressure, 76

U
UF. *See* Ultrafiltration (UF)
Ultrafiltration (UF)
        ADHF, 91–94
        applications
                Aquadex system 100, 102, 103
                cardiac function, 101
                correlation, neurohormone levels, 101
                CVVH, 102

Ultrafiltration (UF) (*cont.*)
    mechanical fluid removal, 100
    neurohormonal levels, 105
    UNLOAD trial, 104
    use, device, 102, 103
  Aquadex system, 106
  congestion, lung
    ACE, 94
    CVP, 94
    GFR, 94
    NSAID, 94
    PCWP, 94–95
    RAP, 94
    renal dysfunction, 95
  diuretic resistance, 98–99
  DRG, 107
  loop diuretics, 95–98

pathophysiology, hypervolemia, 92–94
PRR, 99
RAAS, 99, 100
SCUF, 105
serum creatinine, baseline, 106, 107

V
Val-HeFT. *See* Valsartan in HF Trial
    (Val-HeFT)
VALIANT. *See* Valsartan in Acute
    Myocardial Infarction Trial
    (VALIANT)
Valsartan in Acute Myocardial Infarction
    Trial (VALIANT), 33
Valsartan in HF Trial (Val-HeFT),
    13, 14, 25, 29